Spirituality & Health Care

The *Special Topics in Health and Faith Series* also includes:

Religion and Public Discourse:
Principles and Guidelines for Religious Participants

The Challenges of Aging: Retrieving Spiritual Traditions

Physician Assisted Suicide:
Religious and Public Policy Perspectives

SPIRITUALITY & HEALTH CARE
Reaching toward a Holistic Future

◆

John Shea

Published by

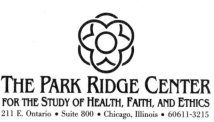

THE PARK RIDGE CENTER
FOR THE STUDY OF HEALTH, FAITH, AND ETHICS
211 E. Ontario • Suite 800 • Chicago, Illinois • 60611-3215

Spirituality and Health Care
Reaching toward a Holistic Future

by John Shea

Research for this book was underwritten by the Fetzer Institute.

Published by   The Park Ridge Center
                 for the Study of Health, Faith, and Ethics
                 211 East Ontario Street, Suite 800
                 Chicago, Illinois 60611

ISBN: 0-945482-02-7
Ethics/Medical/Legal/Religion

Printed in Canada

CONTENTS

INTRODUCTION

A CONVERSATION BETWEEN HEALTH CARE AND SPIRITUALITY

☐ ☐ ☐ ☐

Entering the Room

Imagine this scenario.

A conversation about health care and spirituality is scheduled to take place in a large, well-lit room. The health care side of the conversation has convened this meeting, so the room is in the corporate headquarters of a health care system. This meeting has not been called to make a pressing decision or to engage in strategic planning for the future. Its purpose is to understand the diverse ways health care and spirituality are presently interacting and to find a way to evaluate the mushrooming proposals on how they should interact.

In the area of health care and spirituality something is afoot. Change is in the air. Some of the ferment is coming from medical researchers who have a growing appreciation of religion and spirituality as variables of mental and physical health. Some of it is coming from boards of directors who are concerned with the faith-based identity of specific health care systems. Some of it is coming from doctors and nurses who have pointed complaints about having to conduct their work in such a way that they are losing their soul. Some of it is coming from organizational gurus who are trying to access spirit in the workplace. Some of it is coming from advocates of holistic health. Some of it is coming from ethics committees which are seriously concerned about the wellsprings of moral action. Finally, as might be expected, some of it is coming from pastoral care people who see an expanded role for their knowledge and abilities and are discussing whether to change their department name to "spiritual services."

What is all this about? How should we think about it?

There are two doors into the room where the meeting will be held. All the people whose primary concern is health care will enter through one door. They are physicians, nurses, medical social workers, managers, human resource personnel, information managers, support staff, lawyers, senior management, CEOs, trustees, members of the board of directors, and so forth. They carry an agenda and will come with certain concerns. Of course, one of these concerns is how to assess this recent interest in spirituality. However, this concern is part of a network of concerns. Some of these other considerations are

- patient satisfaction
- excellent medical care

- employee morale
- measurable results
- financial growth
- government regulations
- organizational restructuring
- HMO negotiations
- performance excellence
- new technologies
- a religiously plural workforce and patient population
- mission integration

In the conversation between spirituality and health care, the entire business and vocation of health care is present. Everything is in the room; nothing is left at the door.

Through the second door will enter all those people whose primary concern is spirituality.[1] They have been invited to listen and respond, to bring their knowledge and expertise into dialogue with the emerging interest in spirituality. These people include chaplains, theologians, clergy, spiritual teachers, and congregational ministers of care from the diverse religious communities and traditions of the world. Also, there will be academic representatives—anthropologists, psychologists, sociologists, philosophers, and historians who study religion and spirituality in contemporary settings. Finally, there will be people who have keen interests in spiritual de-

---

1. Imagining the conversation in this "two door" fashion is not meant to give the impression that the health care side is not living a spiritual life day in and day out. Just the opposite. It is presupposed that the spiritual is present and active in the lives and operations of the health care providers. In fact, it is just this awareness of the spiritual life that prompts the need for dialogue with those who are explicitly concerned with spirituality.

velopment but who refuse to identify with detached academic study or with any organized religion.

These three sets of spirituality people are highly diverse and have multiple agendas. However, in general, their role is to retrieve from their personal experience and their intellectual and spiritual traditions whatever will contribute to the conversation. Determining the "whatever" is the key. The spirituality people know about the beliefs, stories, and practices of spiritualities. They have opinions about what counts as spiritual development. They have thought at length about how contemporary culture both blocks and encourages spiritual growth. They have been part of inter-faith dialogues and have developed rules about borrowing beliefs, stories, and practices from traditions that are not one's own. They know the importance, even the necessity, of both spiritual guidance and community support. Yet they also know the dangers of gurus and spiritually based communities. They have theories about how the spiritual influences the physical, psychological, and social. In other words, they are knowledgeable in the area in which health care is interested.

But what of all this—their own knowledge and the wisdom of the traditions they represent—is relevant? What will both affirm and critique the spiritual interest of health care in such a way that new possibilities will be seen? This is what the conversation will determine.

A Love Affair in the Making?

The participants hope the conversation will result in appreciative perspectives and ways of seeing and evaluating the multiple interactions of spirituality and health care. In order for this to happen, the dialogue must be mutual, both sides enriching the other. Whatever the spirituality people have to offer, it cannot be put forward on its own terms and left to stand. Although articulating the dynamics of spiritualities from their own internal viewpoints is important, it is too unrelated and insufficiently tailored to the health care situation. Whatever is said has to be in open dialogue with the societal, organizational, and medical realities of health care.

The same is true for the health care side. Health care cannot put forward its present situation in such a way that it becomes a cookie cutter for every input from the spirituality side. When this happens, any idea that does not fit with current organizational structures or medical assumptions is quickly dismissed. If a perspective is to emerge that will be able to direct, develop, and prune the relationship of spirituality and health care, there must be openness and flexibility in both dialogue partners.

In general, this meeting of health care and spirituality can be seen as a merger of two diverse, yet complementary, levels of existence and two diverse, yet complementary, languages. Health care deals with what blatantly manifests itself in the physical, mental, and social dimensions of people's lives. Its languages are ever in the process of refinement, seeking greater and greater nuance, always analytical, always on the verge of strategy. Spirituality deals with what is hidden to conventional eyes, "a subtle something,"[2] present yet elusive. It senses something essential but invisible. Its primary

2. Jeffrey Levin, "How Prayer Heals: A Theoretical Model," *Alternative Therapies* Vol. 2 No. 1 (January 1996), 66.

languages are imaginative and evocative, seeking to help people recognize the spiritual in their midst. These two languages and the levels of life they express might easily miss one another, each one thinking the other is second best.

Yet health care and spirituality need one another. Their mutual attraction is analogous to the relationship David Whyte sees between the corporate person and the poet.

> The poet needs the practicalities of making a living to test and temper the lyricism of insight and observation. The corporation needs the poet's insight and powers of attention in order to weave the inner world of soul and creativity with the outer world of form and matter.[3]

Health care is a world of practicalities that needs to be in touch with the inner world of soul lest it carry on its tasks in mechanical and dispirited ways. Spirituality points to the human capacity for transcendence and needs to be tested and tempered, in this case by the concrete and practical concerns of health care, lest its dreams of a better world remain dreams. Health care has drawn its symbol of healing—the snake that sheds its skin and becomes new—from Greek mythology. In this contemporary situation, it might return to Greek mythology to learn from Ulysses. Alfred North Whitehead said that Ulysses belonged to the "world of the gods and the world of the foxes." Bringing together the gods and foxes,

---

3. David Whyte, *The Heart Aroused: Poetry and the Preservation of the Soul in Corporate America* (New York: Doubleday, 1994), p. 9.

the spiritual and the practical, is one way of imagining the conversation between health care and spirituality.

Another way of imagining the conversation is to see it as an attempt to make a whole person. The half-person of health care, both organizationally and medically, is characterized as immersed in this world, fighting for survival and position, concerned with measuring the measurable, its nose never lifted from the grindstone. The half-person of spirituality is characterized as otherworldly, blue-sky gazing, tripping over particulars it never notices, unable to seriously value the flesh that fades. These two different half-people are in the same room for a common conversation. From a Buddhist perspective and with different language, John Tarrant articulates the halves' desire to mingle.

Secretly, spirit (the half-person of spirituality) wants embodiment, wants to sink down and be mortal, to bleed, to struggle with high blood pressure and menstrual cramps and cold toes. Without these pains, spirit is ghostlike, vague, adrift without links to the earth. And (the half-person of health care) which knows more than it needs to about the fragility of the body, secretly loves weightlessness, the voice of the soprano, rising like a lark vertically above the tussocks at dawn. We need both realms. We are at once vast and tiny, intensely personal and at peace.[4]

<hr>

4. John Tarrant, *The Light Inside the Dark* (New York: HarperCollins Publishers, 1998), p. 216.

When the conversation between health care and spirituality becomes difficult, it is good to remember their deeper love affair, their desire to supply what is missing in the other, their cooperation in the adventure of human evolution, their fellowship on the journey of walking each other home.

Two Colloquia

The Park Ridge Center and the Fetzer Institute cosponsored two conversations on the relationship of spirituality and health care. Although the participants in the conversation did not match exactly those in the imaginary scenario at the beginning of this introduction, both the health care and spirituality sides of the conversation were well represented.

The first meeting, "Spiritual Resources in Health Care," was held in late May of 1998. At this academic, interdisciplinary meeting, the participants represented perspectives from medicine, medical research, sociology, psychology, anthropology, and theology. The overarching goals of the colloquium were to gain some perspective on the relationship between spirituality and health care and to develop some characterizations of spirituality that would illumine and direct the current interest in spirituality within health care. It was a "big picture" meeting. Some of the ideas from this meeting were developed into articles for the Park Ridge Center's 1998 January/February *Bulletin*, "Spirituality in Health Care."

The second colloquium, "The Practice of Spirituality Within Health Care: The Present and Future State of the Art," was held in June of 1999 and was more practically oriented. The conversation revolved around (1) collecting information on programs and initiatives that are either in place or are being developed around spirituality within health care;

(2) identifying the spiritual-theological, ethical, and organizational issues that are emerging as a result of trying to implement these programs; (3) evaluating what is happening and could happen in the light of the spiritual wisdom of diverse religious traditions as this wisdom is being articulated by contemporary spiritual teachers who themselves may or may not be organizationally connected to health care; and (4) outlining key components of educational and formational strategies for programs on spirituality within health care. If the first colloquium (in the words of one of the participants) was "where the rubber hits the sky," the second colloquium was concerned with "how the rubber hits the road."

In both meetings, the conversations were wide-ranging and collaborative. Although short papers were written and presentations given and responses made to both, the dialogue went beyond this. People spoke from both their professional expertise and their personal experience. What emerged were insights and perspectives that were initiated by individuals but were subsequently refined and reshaped through the affirmations and challenges of conversation.

This book is neither a direct report of those meetings nor a consensus document. The participants at those colloquia are not responsible for the content of these pages. Those conversations simply became the raw material that I have shaped in a certain way. Or, in another metaphor, the ideas were springboards into further considerations. Consequently, I have deselected some thoughts and combined others. Also, I have added material of my own and drawn on insights from other writings. In particular, I have brought forward spiritual wisdom from different religious traditions, wisdom I thought would enrich the conversation by deepening the un-

derstanding of how spiritualities work and what they are
meant to do.

Entering Through the Spirituality Door

At one point the question was asked, "What is everyone
bringing to the table?" That is a good question. It clarifies
where people are coming from and openly acknowledges limits. My own answer to that question is "I come from the spirituality side of the conversation and so enter through the second door." At first I was not sure what a theologian, spiritual teacher, and retreat master like myself could contribute.
In the course of many conversations and much reading, I began to see what I brought to the table and began to wonder
how valuable it was.

Some conversations focused on quantitative research that
showed connections between spiritual beliefs and practices
and the prevention, treatment, coping, and cure of various
diseases. My immediate response was to pursue the inner processes that were presupposed in the data. If Bible reading
helped seventy-to seventy-five-year-old African-American
males cope with coronary artery disease, I wanted to know
what passages of the Bible they were reading. What went on
inside them as they read those passages?

Other conversations dwelt on qualitative studies that encouraged people to tell how their faith influenced how they
thought and acted in health care settings. These studies were
conducted in semistructured interviews, which were then
coded into general categories. Typical examples would be that
spiritualities gave people a sense of "overall meaning" or
"transcendence" or "belonging." My immediate response was

to return to the narrative and the questions that were asked. How does one get at spiritual consciousness? What phrases does one "lift up" and develop from the many pages of narrative? I immediately wanted to extend what the people interviewed were saying, develop it, put it in a larger context that would both affirm and challenge what they said.

Other conversations arose in the context of a commitment to holistic care. People not only talked about physical and mental care but about meeting spiritual needs. A grocery list of spiritual needs was strung together and strategies developed to respond to them. Often chaplains were taken to task for not discerning and working with the spiritual needs of patients and medical caregivers. In these conversations, I always wanted to pursue what a "spiritual need" is. "Need" may not be the best category for talking about the spiritual. The phrase is clumsy and can be taken in the wrong way. Perhaps what sounds like "spiritual need" is really the beginning of spiritual searching. If that is the case, it may be more fruitful to think of what is the next moment of development rather than how to meet a need. Of course, responding to spiritual development entails different practical and theoretical abilities than meeting a need. In general, I was convinced conventional understandings of the spiritual, understandings spiritual teachers often try to dispel, had to be explored more deeply before proceeding further.

Still other conversations focused on the practical matters of education and implementation. If spirituality is important for health care, how can it be included in medical curricula? How can it be integrated into patient care? How can it be recognized and encouraged within the organization? How can it be measured and included in performance evaluations? In these conversations I always felt a need for more "marrow-bone" knowledge. The poet W.B. Yeats wrote

> God guard me from those thoughts men think
> In the mind alone;
> He that sings a lasting song
> Thinks in a marrow-bone.[5]

There seemed to be little intuitive feel for the spiritual. There needed to be more experiential knowledge of the distinctiveness of the spiritual and the peculiar contributions it could make to the health care enterprise. So my general response was always in the direction of greater understanding and more firsthand acquaintance with the reality of the spiritual. This, of course, is not always welcomed in practical and political conversations.

When the spirituality side enters the conversation, there is also a question of language. Many different languages angle into the multiplex world of health care. Most people are comfortable with the languages of medicine, business, law, and organizational development.

When spirituality talks however, there is often a noticeable discomfort. Spirituality often borrows the languages of religious traditions. Words like Spirit, soul, God, sacred, grace, and salvation are on the table. There are also words that have special meaning in the mystical stands of religious traditions— transcendence, communion, interiority, the world, detach-

---

5. *W.B. Yeats: The Poems*, ed. Daniel Albright (J.M. Dent & Sons, 1990), p. 332.

ment, emptiness, and so on. These words and many others often are not immediately understood. Sometimes it is because they belong to one religious tradition, and people from other traditions do not connect with them. At other times, it is because these words refer to ultimate realities, and it is difficult to relate them to the practicalities of health care. At other times, it seems to be just secular embarassment at the whole spiritual project. It is an instance of Flannery O'Connor's observation that the word *God* embarrasses contemporary people in conversation the way the word sex had embarrassed earlier generations.

Whatever the reasons for the discomfort, the language of the spirituality side has to adapt if it is going to be heard. It has to be able to describe the spiritual processes it thinks are central to health care, and it has to be able to describe them so that people who are not fully acquainted with the contemporary cultural language of spirituality or fully socialized into a specific religious tradition can acknowledge them. Spirituality cannot just talk. It has to talk to people who are open to the conversation but who are not willing to be overwhelmed by a technical vocabulary.

Therefore, the contribution from the spirituality side, or at least my contribution from the spirituality side, could be characterized in organizational language as "added value." Something is already afoot. The results of quantitative and qualitative studies are making an impact. There is a widespread commitment to holistic care, a care that includes the spiritual. Education programs are already designed; implementation procedures are in place. The spirituality side begins by listening carefully to what is already happening and finding openings where it can add understanding, information, and material that will be valuable. It listens first, and it talks second. Its purpose is to enhance and build up. However, sustained input from the spirituality side can be more than merely additive. It can reconfigure how the overall project of spirituality and health care is conceived.

This book is written from the perspective of what the spirituality side of conversation can contribute. It tries to look inside the connections the quantitative studies are uncovering, tries to find openings for development in the firsthand accounts of spiritually aware people in health care, explores the distinctiveness of the spiritual, and tries to ground education and implementation efforts in a more profound understanding of spiritual processes. Finally, it attempts to do all this in a spiritually accessible language. This language borrows words from specific religious traditions, but it also includes accompanying language meant to show what the inherited religious language reveals about the spiritual dimension of human experience.

The Structure
This book is what I consider a "middle work." It is not a philosophical or theological treatise that attempts to reconceive the foundations of both health care and spirituality. Neither is it a practical how-to approach, detailing four steps, three prerequisites, and two criteria. It occupies a place between overarching theory and specific practice. This middle position works with observations and ideas that reflect deeper philosophical and theological concerns and simultaneously are important for policies and practices. These observations and ideas provide a way of seeing the territory that is known by the dense code name, "health care and spirituality."

In this code name, both words have to be unpacked. As this book unfolds, the many passageways these two words open up will be traveled. However, at the beginning, it is necessary to say a word about that most elusive of words, spirituality. In much of the literature on health care and spirituality, there is an obsessional quest to define spirituality.[6] At the same time, some observers reluctantly admit there are as many definitions as there are people who use the word. It is alleged that it is easier to nail jello to a tree than to define spirituality.[7]

It seems to me all these definitions are helpful in certain settings. Perhaps a more manageable approach is to forsake the goal of a complete and inclusive definition. Instead, spirituality could be characterized in ways that would be appropriate to its context and its ambitions. Spirituality would be characterized one way within the home territory of a faith tradition, another way when considered in the context of a counseling session, and still another way when used by an organization interested in linking employee morale with increased productivity. What is needed is partial, yet significant, characterizations of spirituality that interact creatively with different contexts. In the case of health care, my suggestion is to break up spirituality into three component

6. For attempts to negotiate the problem of defining spirituality, see Walter Principe, "Toward Defining Spirituality," *Studies in Religion* 12 (1983); Rachel Naomi Remen, "On Defining Spirit," *Noetic Sciences Review* (1998); Robert A. Emmons, *The Psychology of Ultimate Concerns* (New York: Guilford Press, 1999); Ian I. Mitroff and Elizabeth A. Denton, *A Spiritual Audit of Corporate America* (San Francisco: Jossey-Bass Publishers, 1999).
7. Gregory F. Augustine Pierce, "Disciplines for a Spirituality of Work," *Origins 32* (January 1999).

parts— spiritual interests, the spiritual, and spiritualities. The rationale for this approach will unfold in the course of these pages, for these three parts provide the structure for the book.

Part One— "Six Spiritual Interests within Health Care"— outlines the spiritual interests that have arisen within the enterprise of health care. At a minimum, spiritual interest connotes a willingness to investigate, a sense that something important might be present. The dawning of spiritual interest is often accompanied by an inner voice saying, "It's worth a look." (1) Patients hear this voice when they are faced with the prospect of losses and limits and suddenly find themselves reevaluating what is important in their lives. (2) Medical caregivers hear this voice when they hope to facilitate the spiritual resources of patients because it may be an important factor in their patients' health and healing. (3) Medical caregivers hear this voice a second time when they assess what is happening to their vocation as healers in the changing marketplace of medicine. (4) Chaplains hear this voice as a way to develop their traditional concerns, to expand their role within the organization, to connect more effectively with congregational clergy, and to relate to the interfaith populations of both patients and employees. The voice of spiritual interest is also heard (5) in the efforts of the leaders and employees to create a better working life within the organization and (6) in the ongoing ethical struggles that permeate every aspect of health care. In all six of these areas there is an intuitive sense the spiritual should be explicitly present as a resource for what is happening.

Part Two—A Working Knowledge of the Spiritual—focuses on the reality of the spiritual that is the presupposition of the six interests and the ultimate reason why people create and espouse spiritualities. In this way, Part Two provides a philosophical bridge between Part One and Part Three. A working knowledge is not a unified theory. It does not attempt to take everything into account and integrate the diversity through the use of ever more comprehensive concepts. Rather, it is a partial understanding, selecting aspects that seem particularly appropriate to the context under consideration and seem to have practical implications. Working knowledges as such are unfinished, always looking to add an insight or expand in a complementary direction or deal with an implication that was previously unseen. In short, working knowledges are works in progress.

A working knowledge of the spiritual within health care begins by positioning the spiritual as a "new kid on the medical block," a complementary dimension to the already established physical, psychological, and social dimensions. Health care attends to each of these dimensions, both in their distinctiveness and in how they influence one another. Attending to the spiritual is envisioned as an inner journey of awareness into the soul space, a space that both connects with a transcendent source and informs and vitalizes everything in people and in the world. As such, it is a subtle, but powerful, resource for creating organizational and individual responses that better situations. However, staying in touch with this resource is not easy. If that is what is desired, and the emerging spiritual interests of health care seem to suggest it is, that entails welcoming and developing spiritualities, for spiritualities are the beliefs, stories, and practices people use to stay in touch with the spiritual.

Part Three—"Welcoming and Developing Spiritualities"—

explores how the interests (Part One) in the spiritual (Part Two) can be pursued. People enter health care settings with the spiritualities—beliefs, stories, and practices—that have been developed within spiritual communities. The purpose of these spiritualities is to consciously open people to the influence of the spiritual. They are background spiritualities geared mainly to community life. However, there is a need for foreground spiritualities—beliefs, stories, and practices that connect more directly with the daily dynamics of health care. These foreground spiritualities are companions of both organizational and individual values and contribute to their implementation. Therefore, a final section of Part Three will outline some of the beliefs, stories, and practices that seem well matched to the spiritual people who inhabit the social roles of patient, family member, friend, medical caregiver, chaplain, board member, leader, administrative manager, medical manager, and so forth. These spiritualities will be a spirituality of self-remembering, a spirituality of knowledge, and a spirituality of compassion.

"An Afterword: Eight Injunctions" recasts some of the perspectives of the book in the form of spiritual imperatives. Injunctions have an honored place in spiritual traditions. They are meant to send seekers down a path of spiritual discovery, to point them in the right direction. All that will be found cannot be foreseen. The injunction initiates an adventure; it does not prescribe a set of predicatable learnings. If the injunctions are heeded, the wager is they will take people deep into the relationship between spirituality and health care.

This short book on health care and spirituality emphasizes the "and." The conversation hopes to integrate the two sets of concerns. As in any genuine dialogue, both sides are changed in the process of talking to one another. When health care probes its spiritual interests and acknowledges its transcendent longings, its self-sufficiency cracks. It accepts its need for, what William James simply called, the More. When spirituality responds, it reconceives itself in order to effectively interact with health care's spiritual interests. Spirituality no longer looks and speaks like it does within the homeland of specific religious traditions. The dialogue has affected both partners. The conversation is generating a third thing. It goes by the dense code name of "health care and spirituality."

PART ONE

SIX SPIRITUAL INTERESTS WITHIN HEALTH CARE

A Spiritually Interested Culture

Despite frequent comments about secularization in western society and a decrease in church membership, there is widespread evidence of a hunger for the spiritual. . . . [This] interest in spirituality is certainly not confined to churchgoers or those commonly identified as religious people.[1]

1. Philip Sheldrake, *Spirituality and History* (New York: Crossroad, 1992), p. 1.

As John Coleman notes, "It is quite clear that there is, palpably, a large and exploding marketplace for spirituality in America."[2] Other cultural commentators have noted the same emerging spiritual interest, an interest that spans generations.[3] It is present among the elderly,[4] the baby boomers,[5] generation X,[6] and even children.[7] This widespread interest suggests that the image of America is shifting from a secular culture to a spiritually interested culture.

Why is there an exploding interest in the spiritual? Some commentators point to positive influences: contact with Eastern religions and spiritual philosophies, an increase in scientific knowledge that leads into mystery rather than away from it, a mind-boggling awareness of the reach of the cosmos, a deepened sense of our symbiotic relationship with the

2. John A. Coleman, S.J., "Exploding Spiritualities: Their Social Causes, Social Location and Social Divide," *Christian Spirituality Bulletin* (Spring 1997).

3. Phyllis A. Tickle, *Rediscovering the Sacred: Spirituality in America* (New York: Crossroad, 1995); Robert Wuthnow, *After Heaven: Spirituality in America Since the 1950s* (Berkeley: University of California Press, 1998); Don Lattin and Richard Cimino, *Shopping for Faith: American Religion in the New Millennium*; J. Naisbitt and P. Aburdene, *Megatrends 2000* (New York: William Morrow, 1988); Paul Ray, *The Integral Culture Survey: A Study of the Emergence of Transformational Values in America*, (Institute of Noetic Sciences, 1998); Robert K.C. Forman, Kathryn Davision, and Susan Jorgensen, *Grassroots Spirituality* (The Forge Institute).

4. Zalman Schachter-Shalomi and Ronald Miller, *From Age-ing to Sage-ing: A Profound New Vision of Growing Older* (New York: Warner Books, 1995).

5. Wade Clark Roof, A Generation of Seekers: *The Spiritual Journeys of the Baby Boom Generation* (San Francisco: HarperSanFrancisco, 1993).

6. Robert Ludwig, *Reconstructing Catholicism for a New Generation* (New York: Crossroad, 1996); Tom Beaudoin, *Virtual Faith: The Irreverent Spiritual Quest of Generation X* (San Francisco: Jossey-Bass Publishers, 1998).

7. Edwin Robinson, *The Original Vision* (Manchester College, Oxford: The Religious Experience Research Unit, 1977); Robert Coles, *The Spiritual Life of Children* (Boston: Houghton Mifflin, 1990).

earth, a commitment to social justice and the well-being of all people. Welcoming and nourishing these experiences and insights create a spiritual yearning, a intense desire to "be in life in a new way." Diarmuid O Murchu names this yearning as a quest "to reclaim the deep, primal sacred story of our evolving universe; of planet Earth as our cosmic home; in the diverse and magnificent array of life-forms around us; in the largely untold story of the evolution of spiritual consciousness within humanity itself, and, finally, in the contemporary desire to create a one-world family characterized by love, justice, peace, and liberation."[8] Most people could add to this list both personal experiences and other cultural developments that stimulate interest in the spiritual.

Other cultural observers see the interest in the spiritual as a response to negative experiences. People are reaching for the spiritual as a way to reclaim dignity and purpose in the midst of fears, moral failures, and a general sense that "things are out of control." According to these observers, the underlying energy of contemporary spiritual interest is the ambiguous and destructive events of the twentieth century: the ongoing horrors of wars that have demonstrated an increased capacity for violence, runaway technology that dehumanizes people even as it claims to advance their causes, economic uncertainty, terrorism, viral epidemics, increasing disparity between the rich and the poor, moral laxity among the leaders of the world, pervasive narcissism and restlessness, the frantic pace of life, the debunking of the myth of progress, the bankruptcy of a secular point of view, etc.

---

8. Diarmuid O Murchu, *Reclaiming Spirituality* (New York: Crossroad, 1998), p. ix.

Frances Vaughan notes, "In recent travels all over the world I have seen new forms of spirituality appearing everywhere. As people become more conscious that problems such as pollution, overpopulation, war, depletion of resources and the devastation of the planet are human caused, there is a growing awareness of the urgent need for changing human consciousness and behavior."[9] Most people could add to this list both personal experiences and other cultural developments that profoundly worry them, that make them pause and consider the possibility of the spiritual.

Traditionally, both positive and negative experiences have awakened people to the spiritual. Thus, in any given individual, the interest in the spiritual may emerge both as a recoiling response to certain negative experiences and as an inclination to pursue certain positive experiences. The positive and negative work together to stimulate the interest.

As Philip Sheldrake noted in the quotation that opened this chapter, this spiritual interest can be found in the culture at large. It is not confined to churches, synagogues, mosques, and temples. Organized religion may be the home of the spiritual, but it is not its exclusive dwelling place. Interest in the spiritual is emerging in the corporate world; in the athletic sphere; in areas of social justice; in the struggles of community organizing; in the ecological, feminist and elder movements[10]; and, of course, in health care. This widespread interest in the spiritual has spurred some commentators to

---

9. Frances Vaughan, *Shadows of the Sacred* (Wheaton, Il: Quest Books, 1995), p. xv.

10. Confer Roger S. Gottlieb, ed., *A New Creation: America's Contemporary Spiritual Voices* (New York: Crossroad, 1990); Peter Van Ness, ed., *Spirituality and the Secular Quest* (New York: Crossroad, 1996).

understand the spiritual search as an anthropological constant. It is a human birthright, part of the human condition. It can be ignored and dismissed, but it cannot be eradicated. In the past, this spiritual search, which is a potential in every person, was pursued by only a few or restricted to the elite of organized religions. Today many are interested—even if they are interested only on their own terms.

This larger cultural interest in the spiritual is the context for the spiritual interests that are emerging within health care. Health care and the spiritual have always been closely related, in part because health care attends to people as they suffer, and suffering is often a time of spiritual invitation. In times of sickness, people reevaluate their lives and ask questions about what is ultimate and true. By its very nature, health care lives at this juncture of human suffering and spiritual search. Also, many health care organizations were founded by communities of faith and today remain religiously affiliated, so naturally they combined medical and spiritual care, refusing to restrict their attention to only physical and mental health. Today, however, these reasons do not provide a complete explanation for the interest in the connection between health care and spirituality. The larger cultural interest has to be taken into account as the context that encourages the specific spiritual interests of health care. Daniel Sulmasy says it succinctly, "The same spiritual hungers that are affecting the rest of society are affecting health care professionals as well."[11]

---

11. Daniel Sulmasy, *The Healer's Calling: A Spirituality for Physicians and Other Health Care Professionals* (New York: Paulist, 1997), p. 8.

Spiritual Interests and Spiritualities

Whatever the causes of the current hunger for the spiritual, it should be stressed that it is just that—a hunger. It is an interest, an inclination, a sense that the spiritual may be a missing piece. It is an inchoate yearning, a formless reaching out for something that is not explicitly known but sensed as crucial.[12] It is talked about as a desire ("In brief, according to our respondents, spirituality is the basic desire to find ultimate meaning and purpose in one's life and to live an integrated life.[13]) or a need ("The most important thing in defining spirit is the recognition that spirit is an essential need of human nature"[14]). The cultural interest in the spiritual and the way that interest manifests itself in different spheres is a beginning, an initial awakening, a first step on a spiritual journey that has the reputation of taking people places they never dreamed of going.

This spiritual longing naturally unfolds into a spiritual search. People become seekers and create a market for spiritualities. Spiritualities are sets of beliefs, stories, and practices that open up and develop the spiritual interest. They show how the hunger can be fed, how the interest can be pursued. Therefore, the quest for spiritualities is energized

---

12. For the dangers involved in the combination of a spiritually interested culture and a spiritually illiterate culture, see John A. Coleman, S.J., "Exploding Spiritualities: Their Social Causes, Social Location and Social Divide," *Christian Spirituality Bulletin* (Spring 1997). Also, for a profound critique of much of what is passing for spiritual interest, see Ken Wilber, *Eye to Eye: The Quest for the New Paradigm* (Boston: Shambhala, 1990), especially Chapter 8, "The Pre-Trans Fallacy," and *One Taste* (Boston: Shambhala, 1999), pp. 111–112.

13. Ian I. Mitroff and Elizabeth A. Denton, *A Spiritual Audit of Corporate America* (San Francisco: Jossey-Bass Publishers, 1999) p. xv.

14. Rachel Naomi Remen, "On Defining Spirit," *Noetic Sciences Review* (1998): 64.

by the intuitive interest in the spiritual, the desire to follow what at first is only a clue.

This distinction between spiritual interest and spiritualities is important. Spiritual interest always emerges out of particular situations. It has definite expectations, even if those expectations are difficult to articulate. It knows what it wants and what it does not want. In other words, spiritual interest is discriminating; the spiritual hunger is looking for a specific menu. Spiritual interest decides which spiritualities or parts of spiritualities will be adopted and which will not be pursued.

For example, many people immersed in the demands of family and work often feel they are "losing themselves." Their inner sense is that they chop a lot of trees, but they have lost sight of the forest. They are making excellent time, but they have forgotten where they are going. Therefore, they are looking for ways to remember who they are as they do what has to be done. This is their spiritual interest—how to stay in touch with the deeper levels of themselves as they engage the tasks of work and family.

Often these people encounter spiritualities that have been developed in monastic settings.[15] This initial meeting seldom goes well. It is difficult to see how spiritual practices such as silence, fasting, and regular prayer times can fit into realities of life in the world. Also, it is not clear how these practices respond to the particular shape of a spiritual interest. How do they help struggling people stay focused in the midst

---

15. See Gregory F. Augustine Pierce, "Disciplines for a Spirituality of Work," *Origins 32* (January 1999), p. 28.

of the fray? This spirituality does not seem to be sufficiently correlated to the spiritual interest. Perhaps with further exploration this surface mismatch will give way to deeper levels of connection. If this does not happen, the result is, on one hand, a spiritual interest that is not pursued and runs the risk of withering and, on the other hand, a spirituality that cannot adapt to new and challenging situations.[16]

Therefore, it is helpful to inquire more deeply into the spiritual interest. How is the spiritual interest being articulated? What is the context that makes the interest understandable? What is hoped for if this interest is pursued? The answers to these questions determine the shape of the spiritual interest and the exact way it opens to further explorations of the spiritual through specific spiritualities.

The Spiritual Interest and Other Interests

There is a particular need to explore the shape of the spiritual interest within health care as it interacts with other interests. Since health care is not one thing but a confluence of many factors, the spiritual interest will be influenced by other interests—by medical practice, organizational and business concerns, economic realities, governmental regulations,

---

16. The emphasis here is how the spiritual interest becomes a principle of discernment, judging the relevance of existing spiritualities. However, spiritualities—developed ways of thinking and behaving in relationship to the spiritual—also judge spiritual interests. If a spirituality is to have a contemporary audience, it must take into account the particular shape of a spiritual interest. But that does not mean it has to capitulate to it. It can "talk back," showing the inadequacy of the interest or some of its dubious assumptions. The interest has to be honored; it does not have to be worshiped. Matching spiritual interests and spiritualities entails an ongoing dialogue with modifications on both sides.

and insurance practices. The spiritual interest within health care is not pure. It is not emerging from the center of a religious tradition explicitly concerned with the worship of God and the salvation of souls. It is emerging in a workplace. Therefore, it is an interest mixed with other interests.

The language in which the spiritual interest is expressed often reflects this mix of interests.

"Introducing a spiritual screening tool is one way of enhancing customer satisfaction."

"Marketing our faith-based nature will probably increase revenues."

"If we can get the numbers to prove spiritual care decreases hospital stays, we might convince HMOs to pay for it."

"I'm not sure I believe in prayer, but the data says it helps, so I encourage my patients to pray."

"I would like to attend to the whole person as our mission says. Even talk some faith talk. But with the decrease in nursing staff, I have too much basic nursing stuff to do. The system works against our efforts at spiritual care."

The spiritual interest is shaped by all the other interests that pervade health care.

Placing the spiritual interest within this complex of concerns does not mean it becomes a mere instrument, a tool of other purposes, a means to other goals. It is not reduced to a strategy. Harold Koenig makes this point with regard to the mushrooming data on the beneficial effects of religion and spirituality on physical and mental health.

> Becoming religious, only in order to gain positive effects on health, will probably not work very well. Research has shown that persons who use religion as a means to an end do not experience the psychological benefits of religious practice. Rather it is those who involve themselves in religion as an end in itself (i.e., persons with intrinsic faith) who are more likely to experience mental health, greater life satisfaction, and less worry and anxiety.[17]

In a quantitative and qualitative study of business executives, Ian Mitroff and Elizabeth Denton point out the same paradox.

> They (business executives) believed that spirituality is one of the most important determinants of organizational performance. They also believed that people who are more highly developed spiritually achieve better results. In this sense, spirituality may well be the ultimate competitive advantage. However, herein lies a fundamental paradox: those who practice spirituality in order to achieve better corporate results undermine both its practice and its ultimate benefits. To reap the positive benefits of spirituality, it must be practiced for

---

17. Harold G.Koenig, *Is Religion Good For Your Health? The Effects of Religion on Physical and Mental Health* (New York: Haworth Pastoral Press 1997), p. 126.

its own sake. If one practices spirituality without regard to profits, then greater profits can result.[18]

The spiritual coexists with multiple other interests. It interacts with those interests, and those interests may even be furthered by a person becoming more spiritually developed.[19] However, the spiritual is not subservient to the other interests. It is an end in itself.

Although the spiritual is not the servant of organizational and economic concerns, it *is* a companion. In the environment of health care, it may be related to holistic care and increased patient satisfaction, or it may be pushed in a new way into the measurement game, documenting its results in a way that is proper to its particular realm and activity, or it may even enter into how performance excellence is evaluated. Those who think this mixing of spiritual interest with other interests contaminates the spiritual will not be happy. They will attempt to strip away the organizational and financial contexts so that "pure spirituality" can emerge. Those who think this mixture condition obscures the real goals of the health care business will not be happy either. They will attempt to compartmentalize the spiritual and push it to the margins, move it off the organizational chart and connect it with an easily erasable dotted line. Nevertheless, the fact remains that the spiritual interest and the financial and or-

---

18. Mitroff and Denton, *A Spiritual Audit*, xviii.
19. It should be noted, even insisted upon, that pursuing spiritual development often leads people far away from the desire for profits. What looks like a subtle and paradoxical strategy for performance excellence becomes a whole new understanding of what "performance" and "excellence" really mean. Spiritually developed people often become subversive of "business as usual."

ganizational interests live in the same house. They are best explored in terms of how they interact with one another.

Six Spiritual Interests Within Health Care

The interest in the spiritual within health care is actually a matter of many interests. The interest arises in different areas and is shaped by the dynamics of that area. Although it is impossible to name all the areas and the diverse ways the spiritual interest is articulated, it is helpful to distinguish six areas. It is also important not to let these distinctions slip into separations. These areas are intimately connected to one another. Considering them one at a time can deepen the appreciation of each of them, but it should not lead to isolating them from one another. Together they form a network of spiritual interests within health care.

The first and foundational interest in health care inevitably arises in the experience of the patients. In particular, how they and their friends and families face and deal with suffering, loss, and limit. It is important to begin with patients from their own internal point of view. This is their time to enter more deeply into the mystery of health and sickness, to know the truth of W.H. Auden's poem.

> About suffering they were never wrong,
> The Old Masters: how well they
>   understood
> Its human position; how it takes place
> While someone else is eating or opening a
>   window or just walking dully along.[20]

---

20. *W.H. Auden: Collected Poems* (New York Books Vintage International, 1976).

As it is the patient's "turn," so eventually it will be everybody's turn. We are all patients-in-waiting. As patients reach for both medical and spiritual resources, they create the foundational spiritual interest within health care. Every other spiritual interest is in some way related to this first and foremost reality—the human person in the struggles of health and illness.

A second spiritual interest arises among the caregivers—physicians, nurses, social workers, family, friends, and others. Their interest overlaps with the patient's. They want to know how to integrate spirituality into patient care. This interest comes from first-hand experience, but it is also generated by recent research. There is a great deal of interest in measuring the effects of religion and spirituality on physical and mental health. Since medical practice has the reputation of paying attention to evidence, these emerging data have implications for medical education and medical care.

Third, the inevitable flipside of dealing with the spiritual interests of the patient, whether from the patient or caregiver perspective, is to focus on the spiritual interests of the caregivers themselves. Some spiritual teachers would contend that the desire to be open to the spiritual perceptions and questions of another presupposes some conscious contact with one's own spiritual search. Perhaps this has always been part of the inner, motivational world of many caregivers. Now, however, many are asking that it come forward in an explicit way. If they pursue it, caregivers begin to walk a spiritual path, personally developing as they care for others.

The fourth area of spiritual interest emerges among chaplains and pastoral care providers. Helping patients spiritually has always been the responsibility of the pastoral care department. How that spiritual help is construed, however, is changing, especially in the light of interfaith populations. When pastoral care begins to think about itself as spiritual services, it implies a different perspective with new knowledges and abilities. Also, as other sectors of the health care enterprise become spiritually interested, the pastoral care department becomes the most readily available resource. Chaplaincy is still a service based in particular faith traditions, but it is also a service that recognizes and promotes the universal dimension of the spiritual.

A fifth area of spiritual interest emerges within the health care organization itself. Some of this interest is the logical entailment of the spiritual concerns of patients and caregivers. If a health care organization is encouraging these spiritual interests, it must have policies and structures that are friendly to the spiritual. Furthermore, it must extend its spiritual openness toward patients and caregivers to all employees and associates. In some faith-based health care organizations, spiritual sensitivity and spiritual knowledge are included in the criteria for leadership. Spiritual interest in the life of the organization becomes a structural commitment to the spiritual development of everyone from patient to employee.

A sixth area can be found in ethics. Whether a specific action or course of action is ethical is a chronic concern of health care. Some divide this concern into medical, organizational, and "everyday" ethics. Ethical viewpoints are developed for specific medical procedures, for particular organizational policies and modi operandi, and finally for just the general way business and work is carried on. Are the deeper values of the people and the organization manifested in their "everyday" interactions? Ethics becomes spiritually interested when it pursues the personal grounding of human decisions and actions. When it asks how identity, perception, and motivation enter into ethical action, it touches the spiritual. The spiritual interest of ethics involves bringing the person who acts into the center of reflection.

Each of these areas, of course, needs further characterization. In this overview, they cannot be explored in detail. However, we can identify some of their key features. These features will, in turn, be clues to how the spiritual should be understood and what spiritualities will be relevant.

One: The Spiritual Interest of Patients

Susan Sontag has suggested that each person carries two passports, one to the land of the well and one to the land of the sick.[21] Of these two, we only want to use the passport to the land of the well. We resist sickness. It reminds us of our mortality and insists we face questions of loss and limit. When we enter into the health care world as a patient, even if we are in good health, we are often aware of an increased vulnerability. There is an undercurrent of nervousness and fear. The whole environment suggests the precariousness of physical life. Limits are in sight.

Many thinkers associate religion and spirituality with these limit experiences. David Tracy sees limit questions and limit experiences as the way people "open" to the meaningfulness of the dogmas and symbols of revelational religion.[22] Limit

---

21. Susan Sontag, *Illness As Metaphor and AIDS and its Metaphors*. (New York: Doubleday, 1990).
22. David Tracy, *Blessed Rage For Order* (New York: Crossroad, 1975).

experiences put people on the threshold of mystery, a space where, Antonio Machado writes poetically, the soul stays awake, "its eyes wide open/ far off things, and listens/ at the shores of the great silence."[23] In discussing religion, Kenneth Pargament makes the same point.

> Religion generally helps people appreciate what they themselves cannot control. It highlights the limitations of material goods, personal desires, and individual lives. Not only that, it offers a way to come to grip with these limitations . . . Thus it may not be too much of an exaggeration to say that an appreciation for the limits of human agency lies at the heart of religion.[24]

Patients are interested in the spiritual because, simply by being patients, they become aware of loss and limit. They find themselves, often against their wills, listening at the "shores of the great silence."

A number of years ago I was working with older Americans on their spiritual development. The assumption was that even in the midst of physical, mental, and social losses, there may be the possibility of spiritual development. Thus, part of the program involved experimenting with different spiritual exercises. One of these exercises asked the participants to remember three times during the week that they were "children of God" or "made in the image of God." This is a foun-

---

23. Antonio Machado, "Is My Soul Asleep?" in Robert Bly, *The Soul Is Here For Its Own Joy* (Hopewell, N.J.: Ecco Press, 1995).
24. Kenneth Pargament, *The Psychology of Religion and Coping* (Guilford Press, 1997), p. 8.

dational spiritual truth but one that is easily forgotten. The next week they were asked when they remembered this spiritual truth. One woman quietly volunteered, "While I was waiting for the doctor." Everyone nodded. Being a patient pushes our awareness toward the spiritual.

For many patients, this openness to the spiritual is an overt plea for help. It is a search for a cure that doctors may not be able to accomplish or may only be able to accomplish with divine help. It is an attempt to bring the spiritual into the situation in the hope that it will contribute to successful physical and mental outcomes. At other times the openness to the spiritual comes about as patients realize the inevitability of loss and limit. They ask the questions, "How will I "do" with this limit? How will I relate to this loss?" Such questions are reminiscent of Dostoevski's remark, "I pray I may be worthy of my sufferings." Some observers have said that on entering patienthood there is a centrifugal force. So much seems to be moving away from the center of the person who has become a patient. What is sought is a counter force, a centripetal movement that brings things back to the center of the person. The spiritual embodies such a centripetal power. It reestablishes the center of the person who is beset by loss and limit.

John O'Donohue tells the story of a woman facing limit and loss who, with the help of a priest, reestablishes her center, and counters the centrifugal movement with a spiritual centripetal response.

A friend of mine went to the hospital to have a hysterectomy. A priest friend came to visit her on the evening before her operation. She was anxious and vulnerable. He sat down and they began to talk. He suggested to her that she have a conversation with her womb. To talk to her womb as a friend. She could thank her womb for making her a mother. To thank it for all her different children who had begun there. The body, mind and spirit of each child had been tenderly formed in that kind darkness. She could remember the different times in her life when she was acutely aware of her own presence, power and vulnerability as a mother. To thank her womb for the gifts and the difficulties. To explain to it how it had become ill and that it was necessary for her continuing life as a mother to have it removed. She was to undertake this intimate ritual of leave-taking before the surgeons came in the morning to take her womb away. She did this ritual with tenderness and warmth of heart. The operation was a great success. Her conversation with her womb changed the whole experience. The power was not with the doctors or the hospital. The experience did not have the clinical, short-circuit edge of so much mechanical and anonymous hospital efficiency. The experience became totally her own, the leave-taking of her own womb.[25]

Patients are interested in the spiritual because it may hold the secret to how they can relate to their own leave-takings, even the leave-taking of death.

However, there is more. Religious traditions universally suggest that suffering can be a spiritual path. It can take us into the land of Spirit and teach us truths to which we would

25. John O'Donohue, *Eternal Echoes: Exploring Our Hunger To Belong* (New York: Bantam, 1998), pp. 179–80.

not otherwise have access. This is the message John Updike brought back from his fever.

> I have brought back a good
> message from the land of 102 degrees:
> God exists.
> I had seriously doubted it before;
> but the bedposts spoke of it with utmost
> confidence,
> the threads in my blanket took it for granted,
> the tree outside the window dismissed all
>   complaints,
> and I have not slept so justly for years.
> It is hard, now, to convey
> how emblematically appearances sat
> upon the membranes of my consciousness;
> but it is truth long known,
> that some secrets are hidden from health.[26]

The "secrets that are hidden from health" concern the spiritual grounding of life. Updike's sickness became an invitation to explore this previously hidden truth—the mundane obviousness of God. Sickness is a chaotic event on all levels, disturbing physical, psychological, social, and spiritual equilibrium. Yet in many situations, the spiritual disturbance is an invitation to growth, a challenge to greater spiritual realization.

---

26. John Updike, *Collected Poems, 1953–1993* (New York: Knopf, 1993), p. 28.

This seems to be the case with Joan Didion.[27] In her auto-
biographical essay "In Bed", she unfolds her ongoing relationship to her migraine headaches. She has taken up any
number of attitudes toward them. She has denied them,
fought them, and tried to understand them. But now she
thinks she is "wise in its ways."

> I no longer fight it. I lie down and let it happen. At first ev-
> ery small apprehension is magnified, every anxiety a pound-
> ing terror. Then the pain comes, and I concentrate only on
> that. Right there is the usefulness of migraine, there in that
> imposed yoga, the concentration on the pain. For when the
> pain recedes, ten or twelve hours later, everything goes with
> it, all the hidden resentments, all the vain anxieties. The mi-
> graine has acted as a circuit breaker, and the fuses have
> emerged intact. There is a pleasant convalescent euphoria. I
> open the windows and feel the air, eat gratefully, sleep well. I
> notice the particular nature of a flower in a glass on the stair
> landing. I count my blessings.

The sickness has become a yoga, purging her and bringing
her to gratitude, a gratitude that might not be available without the discipline of the migraine.

One of the foremost spiritual invitations that arises from
sickness is to reconcile from the heart. Sickness forces a scru-
tiny, an inward glance into the heart to discern what must
be done. It encourages a process of prioritization. What is
important? The result of this "taking stock" is often the re-

---

27. Joan Didion, *The White Album* (New York: Simon and Schuster, 1979)
p. 172.

alization that words of love have not been spoken. Too much has gone unsaid. Too much has been taken for granted. Under the pressure of illness words of love are spoken, sometimes initiated by the sick and sometimes by the well. These words of love from the heart reestablish broken relationships and revitalize dormant relationships. At the prospect of limit and loss, there is an encouragement for people to reach out to one another. Their essential closeness comes to the surface, breaks through silence into speech.

When the spiritual interest of patients is characterized as the ability to relate to loss and limit and the courage to follow loss and limit into profound spiritual realizations, what spiritualities—beliefs, stories, practices—will critique and develop that interest?

Two: The Spiritual Interest of Medical Caregivers in Patients

"Caregivers" is a broad category. It includes doctors, nurses, social workers, family, friends, visitors, and others.[28] Often these people have specific areas of care. Doctors and nurses, for instance, attend to aspects of physical health and illness; social workers attend to various social contexts; family and friends provide emotional and personal support. These different focuses generate a system of referrals whose goal is to give specialized, quality care to the patient.

However, this division of labor is not absolute. Caregivers find themselves in the presence of the whole person. This person of the patient is always the ultimate subject of care

---

28. Chaplains, congregational clergy, and various ministers of care are certainly caregivers. However, their interest in the spiritual will be considered under the "chaplain" category.

and so what is important to the patient becomes important to the caregiver. The foundational reason for this is that caring for patients means acknowledging and addressing their concerns. Even if the caregiver is a doctor or a nurse, when the patient talks about prayer or God or forgiveness, the conversation is engaged.[29] Daniel Sulmasy thinks that "the fact that religion is important to patients seems to be justification enough" to pursue conversations about spirituality.[30]

Recently, medical caregivers have also found additional reasons for engaging in spiritual conversations with patients. There has been considerable research into the connection between religion, spirituality, and health. A multitude of studies have linked religion and spirituality to specifically medical goals. In general, these studies have shown that religion and spirituality have positive effects on physical and mental health.[31] Although there are methodological questions about this research and ethical questions about its implications, religion and spirituality have become variables in the quest for a better understanding of disease and health.[32]

When religion and spirituality appear on the medical screen in this way, they do so in terms of medical values. These values prize clear definitions, sharp distinctions, and empirical ways to measure results. The exact pathways that religion and spirituality move along to contribute to better

---

29. See Constance Harris Sumner, BSN, RN, OCN, "Recognizing and Responding to Spiritual Distress," *AJN* (January 1998).

30. For an extended discussion of this, see Sulmasy, *Healer's* chapter four: "God-Talk at the Bedside."

31. See Koenig, *Is Religion Good for Your Health?* Dale Matthews, M.D. with Connie Clark, *The Faith Factor: Proof of the Healing Power of Prayer* (New York: Viking, 1998).

32. See R.P. Stone, E. Bagiella, T. Powell, "Religion, Spirituality, and Medicine," *The Lancet* (February 1999): 664–67.

health are probed in the hope they can be consistently traveled. This new appreciation of religion and spirituality moves them from an important but concomitant concern to a potential medical resource in the struggle for health.

Many see this inclusion of the spiritual in medical treatment as part of a history of expansion. Once medical care was narrowly focused on the health and disease of the body. Then the mind was included because of the influences of mental states on the entire organism. Then it was recognized that social factors were crucial determinants of health and disease. Finally, the spiritual and its impact have entered into the purview of the medical approach. The result is a more inclusive picture of what makes for health and sickness, a careful attending to the complete person in his or her physical, psychological, social, and spiritual aspects.[33]

This connection between religion, spirituality, and health raises questions about how doctors are educated and what is the scope of the physician-patient relationship. A growing number of medical schools are now finding space in their curriculum for a course on religion and spirituality.[34] Also, some thinkers encourage physicians to support a patient's spiritual and religious beliefs. This support may include spiritual screening,[35] a basic respectfulness and openness to con-

---

33. See *Piecing Together the Puzzle: The Future of Health and Health Care in America* (Institute for the Future).

34. Christian M. Puchalski, MD, MS, and David B. Larson, MD, MSPH, "Developing Curricula in Spirituality and Medicine," *Academic Medicine*, 73, no. 9 (September, 1998); Howard Silverman, "Creating a Spirituality Curriculum for Family Practice Residents." *Alternative Therapy 3* (1997): 54–61.

35. From a chaplaincy perspective see "Symposium: Screening for Spiritual Risk" *Chaplaincy Today* 15 (1999).

versations about religion and spirituality, and referrals to people more qualified in the area of spirituality.[36] It may also, under certain circumstances, go beyond these. Physician and patient may engage in a common religious practice, for example, attend a worship service together or pray with one another.

These developments raise many theological and ethical questions. Although spiritual activity may enhance mental and physical health, is that what spirituality is about? Or does the spiritual life have to be pursued in terms of its own goals—a deepened relationship to Spirit—and not in terms of its medical effects? In the immediate past a medical caregiver's faith and spirituality were deep background to his or her practice. Does bringing it to the foreground in a noncoercive way require a new set of skills? What type of knowledge of religion and spirituality is necessary in order to be respectful of a patient's faith? If medical caregivers move in this direction, do they enter the arena of symbolic healing where the inner attitudes and the quality of the relationship between physician and patient are paramount? How are the boundaries of medical disciplines respected as inquiry into spiritual concerns and issues are pursued? Can medical caregivers be sensitive to the spiritual concerns of a patient if they themselves are spiritually unconcerned? Do medical

---

36. For the many nuances to this complex issue of physician-patient relationships and conversations about the spiritual, see Larry Vandecreek, "Should Physicians Discuss Spiritual Concerns With Patients?" *Journal of Religion and Health* 38 (Fall 1999). For a number of different perspectives on integrating spirituality into patient care, see *Integrating Spirituality Into Treatment: Resources for Practitioners*, ed. William R. Miller (American Psychological Association, 1999).

caregivers see their practice of medicine as a path of spiritual development for themselves? What ethical and legal questions are involved in this expansion of the medical caregiver's role?

When the spiritual interest of caregivers in patients is characterized as attention to the whole person with a special recognition that the spiritual may have beneficial impact on physical and mental health, what spiritualities—beliefs, stories, practices—will critique and develop the interest?

Three: The Spiritual Interest of Medical Caregivers in Themselves

A question that is often asked in reflection groups of medical caregivers is, Why did you go into health care? The responses vary, but almost all reach beyond the professional into the personal world of relationships and meaning. Some talk about a childhood experience of living in a house with a chronically sick person. Others talk about an experience of being ill and being compassionately cared for by a doctor or nurse. Or they may talk about coming from a family with many nurses and physicians and hearing the same call. Herbert Benson's opinion is frequently confirmed: "physicians often come into medicine to help people because of spiritual beliefs."[37] Often some of these beliefs have to do with themselves. The caregivers see themselves as hearers of a call, a call that arises out of their own talents and desires but also has a transcendent source.

37. Beth Baker, "The Faith Factor: An Interview with Herbert Benson," *Common Boundary* (July-August 1997): 24.

However, it is difficult to maintain this sense of call. The work of health care professionals is besieged by pressures that turn the call into a career and the career into a job. When we see what we do as a career, we have tapped into achievement motivation. We are intrinsically driven to do excellent work and to be rewarded for it. But the bigger picture is lacking; the outward sense of service has been replaced by an inner drive to become the best and to be known for it. And when our career peaks, what we do is in danger of becoming a job. When we do a job, we do it for still other reasons. We often work at jobs for extrinsic reasons, usually financial considerations. The higher calling has then devolved into a money game. This occupational hazard, the slide from calling to career to job, is an inner movement, an attitudinal shift that often occurs before people are aware of it. They only recognize what has happened in hindsight.

All work faces the temptation to be alienated, to be separated from the deeper levels of the self and reduced to numbing, repetitious activity, to fall into the category of "a job" in which there is only limited investment. However, with the multiple changes in the surface structures of health care delivery, the work of physicians and nurses is under particular pressure, a pressure that puts so much emphasis on the "letter" that it kills the "spirit."

Health care professionals used to be awash in abbreviations and acronyms of their own creation: COPD, MI, PT/PTT, CMV, WNL, CBC, and so forth. Now they are drowning in a new set of abbreviations created by others: HMO, PPO, IPA, RBRVS, PPRC, HCFA, and so forth. Specialists are being made into generalists. Generalists are being made into gatekeepers. Hospitals are closing. Practices are being bought. Report cards are being issued. Utilization reviewers scrutinize clinical decisions from a thousand miles away.[38]

It is in this context of increasing clutter and change that many fear something essential is being lost.

If patients are interested spiritually because they have to deal with limit and loss and medical caregivers are interested in patient spirituality because they value holistic approaches and recognize that the spiritual may have beneficial effects on bodily and mental health, then medical caregivers are interested in their own spirituality because they want to maintain or reclaim their sense of vocation. They can do this in many ways. The classic practices of spiritual renewal are retreats, prayer, spiritual reading, and participation in the rituals of a religious tradition. However, these are all activities outside work. What caregivers want is a vocational renewal that will happen in the middle of their work, in their relationships with staff and patients. The same situations that drain them can then become the situations that inspire them.

Relationships are the key. In an interview with selected family practice physicians, the physicians noted that "spirituality was often experienced in the context of relationships with patients."[39] Sulmasy agrees, "The spiritual doctor or nurse or other health care professional is one who enters into relationships of trust with patients: inviting trust, behaving

---

38. Sulmasy, *Healer's Calling* 8.
39. Frederic C. Craigie, Jr. and Richard F. Hobbs, III, "Spiritual Perspectives and Practices of Family Physicians With an Expressed Interest in Spirituality," *Family Medicine* (in press).

in a trustworthy manner regardless of whether of not that trust is reciprocated, and trusting in the basic goodness of a world of healing relationships."[40] On one level the relationship of caregiver to cared for is unequal. The caregiver provides services to the patient. However, there are moments when this dynamic is reversed.

> A second oncology nurse tell the story of the elderly, poor, Hispanic man, whose cancer was beyond any hope of treatment or remission, who came to the nursing station at the end of the day, "long after the doctors had left." He went to each of the staff members, shaking their hands and thanking them for "treating him like a man." The nurse's comment was that this episode helped her, and challenged her, to remember why she was doing what she was doing.[41]

Within such relationships the spirit is touched and the vocation is renewed.

In a vocation of service and giving, it is the sudden and unexpected receiving that often brings renewal.

> You walk the halls of this place, and what do you see from room to room? Most people peer in and see this retarded child or that one. They focus on this particular mannerism or that deformity. I do it too. It's very compelling, that picture.
>
> But one kid flipped me around on that. We were doing

---

40. Sulmasy, *Healer's Calling* 31.
41. Frederic Craigie, "The Spirit and Work: Observations About Spirituality and Organizational Life," *Journal of Psychology and Christianity* 18 (1999).

language exercises. And for some godforsaken reason I'd chosen the exchange "How are you?" . . . "I'm doing fine." We'd go back and forth. Well, he was having quite a hard time of it, slurring out. "Iy dluee fie" or some such. "Let's try again, really slowly," I said. "How . . . are . . . you?" And he slurred, "Iy dluee fie." Then he suddenly burst into this wonderful crazy slurry laugh. It was the nuttiest sound we'd ever heard, either of us. He wasn't doing fine at all. Neither was I. We were doing terribly. It was absurd. We just began to howl.

In the midst of that he suddenly gave me this very clear look—the eyes behind the expression. And I had a sudden thought: "My God, he knows more than I'll ever know about all this. He sees the whole situation." At which point he just scrunched up his face like a clown and gave me this wonderful wink.

I was just stunned. All I could see was this incredible sense of the humor of things. It was so deep in him. He just had it all in perspective. And he gave that perspective to me.

When I left him, my head was spinning. I walked down the hall and looked into the other rooms, at kids I'd known, or so I'd thought, for months. It was totally new. I don't quite know how to describe it. In this room I saw courage. In that room I saw joy. Across the hall, patience. In yet another room, such sweetness: a little body who was so continuously filled with love, people would just—"die," I was going to say. "Live," really.

I felt so humbled. I swear I had the impulse to go down on my knees. Here I was, going around giving speech therapy, little lessons, little tips. And what was I receiving back in return? Humanity. Basic humanity. The deepest qualities of a person, deeper than you'd see most anywhere.

What a gift! How much it helped me in my work! In fact it really changed my life. How often can you say that?[42]

The caregiver on one level becomes a receiver on another level. Experiences such as this make people aware of a dynamic flow of spirit that is deeper than the physical categories of sick and well and the social categories of helper and helpee. These experiences renew people in the midst of work and remind them they are engaged in a vocation.

When the spiritual interest of caregivers in themselves is characterized as renewing their original sense of call by finding spiritual substance in their relationships with patients, what spiritualities—beliefs, stories, practices—will critique and develop this interest?

Four: The Spiritual Interest of Chaplains

The spiritual interest of chaplains is a continuation, a nuancing, and an extension of their perennial concern. Although chaplains wear many hats, attending to the spiritual life of patients has always been important.[43] As Gordon J. Hilsman notes, "Chaplains have developed skills to assess and activate people's spiritual resources during difficult times. They have helped people cope, adjust, accept, and integrate loss and change into the evolving fabric of their lives. They

---

42. Ram Dass and Paul Gorman, *How Can I Help?* (New York: Knopf, 1985), pp. 140–42.

43. Don S. Browning "Hospital Chaplaincy As Public Ministry," *Second Opinion* 1 (1986). Browning characterizes chaplaincy as a public ministry in the service of health. In pursuit of this value, the chaplains functioned as value-committed cultural anthropologists, negotiators of world views, stimulators of ethical deliberation, and stimulators of spiritual growth.

have listened and prayed with people in distress, teased out grief that needed expression, used rituals for healing, and advocated for better or more appropriate care."[44] This personal presence is the classical role of the chaplain, a task that will always be needed.

The knowledge and skills needed to be present to people in this way were often a combination of psychological dynamics and theological content. On the one hand, it was not enough merely to call upon comforting beliefs or engage in prayer. Faith and religious practice had a goal. They were to open people to the Divine Source. Therefore, what was important was how the beliefs and prayers were functioning in the mind of the patient. The psychological reception of faith convictions and practices had to be considered. Faith, by itself, was only half the picture. On the other hand, a strictly psychological approach was important but insufficient. Attending to the mental and emotional climate of the patient, friends, and family left out the deeper theological level, a level that the experience of illness was inviting into awareness. Therefore, the chaplain's task of being present to people meant bringing together psychological sophistication with theological depth.

The current interest in spirituality develops this partnership of psychology and theology. Spirituality is concerned with consciousness and so taps into psychological considerations. But it is especially concerned about moments of transcendent awareness, and so it incorporates theological depth.

---

44. Gordon J. Hilsman, "Competencies of the New (and Some Old) Spiritual Care Work," *Caregiver Journal* 12, (1996): 3.

Spiritual development focuses on times when people sense they are more than the circumstances that envelop them and perceive they are grounded in an ultimate reality. These moments are usually fleeting. Through spiritual practices, this fleeting moment is remembered and brought forward. So the state of consciousness at one moment becomes a trait of consciousness. As a trait of consciousness, it is continually present and can be called upon in stressful and difficult times. Also, the resources of a faith tradition—scripture, rituals, prayers, creeds, and so forth—are evaluated in terms of their potential to facilitate spiritual consciousness. When spirituality is considered in this way, it reflects the type of care that chaplains have always thought to be important.

Another traditional aspect of chaplaincy training and experience has been self-knowledge. In order to be effective with patients, families, and friends, chaplains looked inward to discover their personal styles and their theological convictions. What was the faith that drove them, and how was that faith mediated by their personalities? This project dovetails with the inner orientation of spiritual development. Spiritual development suggests that a person first uncovers the working of God in his or her own life before they try to help others open to the spiritual. As Confucius says in the classic story, "The Fasting of the Heart," "The sages of old first sought Tao in themselves, then looked to see if there was anything in others that corresponded with Tao as they knew it."[45] The inner journey of chaplains is not only a task of self-

---

45. *The Way of Chuang Tzu*, trans. Thomas Merton (New York: New Directions Publishing 1969). Reprinted and commented on in John Shea, *The Legend of the Bells and Other Tales* (Chicago, Il: Acta Publications, 1996), pp. 21–28.

discovery but a path of spiritual development, a path that is nurtured by the ongoing experiences of their chaplaincy.

One such experience, an experience bursting with spiritual potential, is Doug's tale.

The group of chaplain residents in our clinical pastoral education center had been asked to present a pastoral event that seemed to be full of meaning and in some way evocative of theological reflection. The event that Doug shared involved a baby who had been stillborn. The parents wanted to have a memorial service in the hospital chapel. Doug tried in vain to get a more experienced chaplain to officiate at the service because he felt he did not know what to do.

When Doug found that he would need to do the service himself, he quickly prepared some things to say. However, when the nurse brought the stillborn baby into the chapel where he and the parents were, Doug found that he could not say what he had planned to say.

"All I could to was stand there and cry," he said.

Not knowing what to expect, Doug was not surprised when the nurse handed him the baby to hold.

"I want you to baptize my baby," the mother said.

Doug nodded, but he saw no water with which to baptize the baby. Almost without thinking, Doug took a tissue, wiped the tears from the eyes of the parents and his own eyes, and touched it to the baby's head and whispered, "Nicole, I baptize you in the name of the Father, Son and Holy Ghost.[46]

---

46. Told in John Patton, *From Ministry to Theology* (Nashville, Tenn.: Abingdon Press, 1990), p. 11.

Moving experiences like this that are told in story form have always been grist for personal exploration and theological reflection. The agenda of spiritual development approaches these stories in a complementary but slightly different way.

Spiritual wisdom often points to a level of knowing deeper than the rational and its corresponding dependence on skills that have been previously tested. Doug "backed into" a spiritual way of being present, a way of not-knowing that allowed him to open into Mystery and respond in ways that the moment provided. This experience is a milestone on Doug's spiritual path, a path that will inform and transform his chaplaincy. A focus on the spiritual promises to deepen the process of self discovery through reflection on experience.

Chaplains are interested in the spiritual because it develops trajectories already present in their work. But once the spiritual is attended to and reflected on, it points out new areas and suggests new projects. First, the spiritual is not reserved for the crisis moments of life when the physical or mental collapses. It is meant to enhance total well-being. In other words, it is more than a coping mechanism. It is a factor in maintaining health and preventing disease. This wider understanding of the relationship of the spiritual to health has implications for chaplains. Perhaps they need to be in closer collaboration with congregations, parishes, synagogues, and mosques. Together chaplains and congregational clergy need to reclaim their spiritual heritage in terms of what it offers to the experiences of health and disease.

Second, with the emerging interests in the spiritual within health care, chaplains may have new audiences (or old audiences in a new way). Chaplains are the closest and most accessible spiritual resources in health care organizations. As medical caregivers and the organization as a whole become spiritually interested in a new way, chaplains will be called upon. Most likely, it will entail working with groups instead of providing one-to-one personal counseling. Also there will be a need for working knowledge of spiritualities and how they can be welcomed and developed in the hustle and bustle of the health care world. Widespread spiritual interest translates into opportunity, and opportunity translates into challenge.

Finally, and perhaps most urgently, chaplains are spiritually interested because it provides a way to relate to the exploding interfaith population. The traditional ways of pastoral care need to be rethought and expanded in the face of Christian, Jewish, Islamic, Hindu, and Buddhist patients and employees. The spiritual, as it is coming to be used, is the broadest category. It is able to acknowledge and appreciate the diverse perspectives of the various religions of the world. In this interfaith world, chaplaincy is often understood as spiritual care. "Spiritual care" reconceptualizes the role of chaplains and lays out a monumental task. How it will be developed is a complex and difficult challenge.

When the spiritual interest of chaplains is characterized as enhancing their psychological and theological care, affirming and deepening their emphasis on self-knowledge, and showing them a way forward in terms of new alliances, new audiences, and new roles, what spiritualities—beliefs, stories, and practices—will develop and critique that interest?

Five: The Spiritual Interest in Organizational Life

The spiritual interest within the organizational life of health care institutions is logically tied to the medical spiritual interest. If the health care organization is committed to delivering holistic care, a care that encompasses the physical, mental, social, and spiritual aspects of being human, then it also should be interested in the physical, mental, social, and spiritual health of its employees. It would be contradictory to try to deliver spiritual care in a spiritually uncaring environment, to try to give to others what has not been given to you. Therefore, the organization as a whole must include the spiritual in how it attends to its employees if it hopes they will be spiritually sensitive to one another and to the various clientele they serve. William J. Bazan and Daniel Dwyer note that "High quality services cannot be delivered by organizations or people who are not spiritually grounded. . . . Burnout distances caregivers from the recipients of their care, and the entire organization must be committed to employees' spiritual needs to assist in preventing these negative responses." The organizational interest in the spiritual well-being of its employees is part of its mission of holistic care.

In and of itself an organization cannot create people's spiritual beliefs and spiritual sensitivity. But it can be supportive of the resources that a person brings to work. It can cultivate and elicit the spiritual consciousness and motivation that is already there. The supposition is that people have an essential spiritual aspect and they are encouraged and satisfied when that side of them is recognized and invited into the workplace. An organization that is spiritually interested understands this deeper level of people, what Abraham Maslow called "the farther reaches of human nature." It searches out ways to "tap"[47] into it.

---

47. See Jard Kass, "Tapping Into Something Greater Than Ourselves," *Spirituality & Health* (Fall, 1996).

The spiritually interested organization uses motivational techniques that go beyond financial incentives and fear of punishment. It cultivates the personal desires to grow intellectually and to create new ways of doing things. Workers are respected not only because respect might contribute to productivity, but also because respect is an abiding characteristic of the organization's identity. It is the way a spiritually interested organization acts. Such an organization also continually keeps in view the larger meaning of services and products. It is not just what workers do but how what they do contributes to society and, even, enters into and extends God's activity in the world. Paradoxically, when ultimate meanings are present, there is increased attention to detail.

Advocate HealthCare, a faith-based organization sponsored by the Evangelical Lutheran Church in America and the United Church of Christ, provides an example of keeping the big picture in view. It recently drafted "Advocate as Faith-based: A Renewed Focus," a document that outlines seven areas where the faith-based nature of Advocate is visible. One area situates the enterprise of health care in the largest possible context:

Faith-based must include both relatedness to God and responsiveness to the contemporary situation. In other words, there is a transcendent (God-related) aspect to Advocate's identity and an engaged (world-related) aspect.

When we understand ourselves as related to the God, we know that our health care mission does not come primarily from ourselves or even from the immensity of human need. We are listening and responding to a Divine call that is creating passions in us to alleviate, accompany and transform human suffering. This transcendent aspect of our identity means the major changes of contemporary health care do not totally define us. Who we are is always deeper than what is happening.

When we understand ourselves as engaged, the whole panorama of health care in America comes into view. We are listening and responding to cultural images, societal policies, business concerns, medical knowledge, organizational issues. We realize the Divine call to care is carried out in a limited and often resistant world. This means we must be competent, savvy, entrepreneurial and creative. This engaged aspect of our identity means that struggle is essential to who we are. We are always looking for a better way to mediate Divine care into human health and suffering. We humbly recognize that as a health care system seeking to be faithful to a Divine call, we are in ongoing need of growth and change in order to carry out our mission.[48]

Whenever it is possible, a spiritually interested organization places human effort in an ultimate context.

The organizational interest in the spiritual is concerned not only with the whole person of the employee but with the leader's ability to manage change. Health care in America is a rapidly changing enterprise in a highly competitive marketplace, and leaders must be able to evaluate and respond to these changes. The alternatives are often starkly stated: either be able to learn and adapt or be prepared to disappear. The survivors will be those who navigate the currents and not

---

48. *Advocate as Faith-based: A Renewed Focus.* (Oakbrook, Il: Advocate Health Care).

those who either ignore or resist them. In this situation, the abilities that are needed go beyond financial management and technical organizational skills. They are rooted in the person of the leaders, in the inner work they have done with themselves.[49] Some of these abilities are connected with spiritual development—capacities for discernment, compassion, commitment, vision, vulnerability, and grief.[50] Spiritually grounded leaders might be what the times demand.

For example, Peter Senge sees personal mastery as a crucial component of a learning organization. He characterizes personal mastery as a discipline of "continually clarifying and deepening our personal vision, of focusing our energies, of developing patience and of seeing reality objectively."[51] Senge acknowledges the roots of this discipline are in the Eastern and Western spiritual traditions. In a similar vein, Alan Briskin sees the key to organizational learning and adaptive behavior as the ability to see the whole.[52] This capacity to see the whole is directly related to the soul and its development. Without the abilities of the soul, organizations are reduced to piecemeal analyses and bumbling interventions. Spiritually developed people have capacities that are needed to survive and flourish in the changing marketplace.[53]

49. Parker Palmer, *Leading From Within: Reflections On Spirituality and Leadership.*

50. Cf. Gerald A. Arbuckle, S.M., P.H.D., "Mergers in Health Care" *Human Development* 20, no. 2 (Summer, 1999): 42–48.

51. Peter Senge, *The Fifth Discipline: The Art and Practice of the Learning Organization* (New York: Doubleday, 1990), p. 7.

52. Alan Briskin, *The Stirring of Soul in the Workplace* (Berrett-Koehler, Inc.1998). Especially, chapters 1,2, 3.

53. Emilie Griffin, *The Reflective Executive: A Spirituality of Business and Enterprise* (Crossroad, 1993); Eric Klein and John B. Izzo, *Awakening*

Recently, Partners for Catholic Health Ministry Leadership has updated a competency model for leadership that was developed by the Catholic Health Association of the United States (CHA) in 1994.[54] This model has a competency cluster entitled "Vocation." It includes the two competencies called "Spiritually Grounded" and "Integrity." Spiritually grounded leaders have the ability to call upon "the spiritual resources of the Catholic faith tradition, their own personal faith and the faith of their co-workers." Integrity consists in acting on one's values and taking risks consistent with those values. These two competencies combine to suggest a spirituality that is geared to put faith into action, to bring spiritual depth to the pressing problems of change.

This interest in spirituality and leadership is particularly important for faith-based health care. The mission statements of faith-based health care are written from explicitly religious perspectives. The inevitable next step question is, How is this ultimate, religious perspective embodied in concrete organizational structures and specific programs? When a mission statement proclaims it is "continuing the healing ministry of Jesus Christ" or it sees people as "the image of God" or it "welcomes all people as a sign of God's universal care," it is articulating the ultimate context of its activities. How does

Corporate Soul (Fairwinds Press, 1998); David Whyte, *The Heart Aroused: Poetry and the Preservation of the Soul in Corporate America* (New York: Doubleday, 1994); Jack Hawley, *Reawakening the Spirit In Work: The Power of Dharmic Management* (Berret-Koehler Publishers, 1993).

54. "Seeking Leaders for the Future: An Interview with John J. Fontana" *Health Progress.*(May-June, 1999): 50–51. For the original model, see John Larrere and David McClelland, "Leadership for the Catholic Health Ministry," *Health Progress*, (June, 1994): 28–33.

this context make a difference? How does it influence human resources, finance, marketing, ethics, medical practices, and more? This is the ongoing endeavor of mission integration, of bringing all aspects of the organization into alignment with its ultimate vision and deepest purpose.[55]

When spiritual interest arises in patients, medical caregivers, employees, and leadership, it provides a natural and unforced link to the mission statement. Mission statements are always unique appropriations of a faith tradition in the light of its health care mission. However, no matter how diverse mission statements are, cultivating spirit can always be construed as part of their purpose. The underlying rationale is persuasive: "Because we are a faith-based health care organization, we attend to the spiritual interests of patients, the spiritual life of medical caregivers, and the spiritual resources of all employees, especially key leadership." The religious foundation of the organization acknowledges and responds to spiritual interest as one way of carrying out its mission. This becomes a way of bridging the gap between mission statements and practices.

When the spiritual interest in organizational life is characterized as encouraging the deeper level of employees, as focusing on the spiritual abilities of leaders to manage change, and as promoting mission integration, what spiritualities—beliefs, stories, practices—will critique and develop this interest?

---

55. On the relationship between the ultimate and particular in the development of health care leadership, see John Shea, "Challenges and Competencies: The Theological and Spiritual Aspects of Catholic Health care Leadership," *Health Progress* (January-February, 2000).

Six: The Spiritual Interest Of Ethics

Every aspect of health care needs to be approached from an ethical point of view. There are ethical reflections and guidelines around medical procedures, patients' rights, business conduct, and a whole array of organizational issues, from hiring to severance. Consequently, there is also a need to think ethically about new initiatives in the area of spirituality. As medical caregivers ask questions about patient spirituality and religiousness and organizations try to encourage the deeper levels of employees and leaders, the usual range of ethical issues will emerge. There will be questions of confidentially, autonomy, truth-telling and deception, privacy, harassment, fraud, minimizing harm, and accreditation. If physicians are convinced that prayer will help the healing process, should they advocate it to their patients? Should medical caregivers pray for patients without telling them? Are spiritual screening tools in general or some spiritual screening tools in particular an invasion of privacy? As changes are introduced, the everyday practice of medicine and organizational procedures will have to be evaluated in terms of their ethical implications.

Ethics is also interested in spirituality because it enters into and shapes decision making and how those decisions will be carried out.[56] Brian O'Toole has described four ways people approach ethics in health care settings. Some people work primarily (1) from principles or (2) in the light of consequences. Other people ground ethical action in (3) the char-

---

56. See "Integrating Spiritual Values and Beliefs into Ethical Decisionmaking: Challenges and Strategies for Institutional Ethics Committees, " *Ethical Currents* no. 57 (Spring, 1999).

acter of the person acting or (4) in the feelings associated with the action. These diverse approaches are part of the observed way people think and act morally. [57]

However, a spiritual-theological dimension can be present in any of these approaches. The principles can be grounded in theological beliefs; the consequences can be evaluated in terms of religious values; the character that is adhered to can be a spiritual identity that will not be compromised; or the moral feelings may be a tip-off to deeper levels of the heart, levels that have been developed through years of spiritual practice. If a person is religious-spiritual, this dimension most likely will influence their moral decisions. This is especially true in end-of-life care. At that time, religious beliefs about life, death, and afterlife become explicit players in difficult decisions. Ethics is interested in spirituality because it is influential in how people think and act morally.[58]

These concerns of ethics with spirituality are complemented by the interest "everyday ethics" has in spirituality. Everyday ethics does not focus on crunch decisions but on the ability to consistently act on deeper values, especially when the environment does not support those values. It is one thing for an organization to have a series of values—for example, respect for the person, compassion, service to the poor, and excellence. It is quite another thing for the employees of that organization, from corporate leadership to clini-

---

57. Brian O'Toole, "Four Ways People Approach Ethics," *Health Progress* (November-December,1998):. 38–43.

58. For an attempt to combine the spiritual process of discernment with the difficult ethical decisions that surround seriously ill newborns, see Michael R. Panicola, "Discernment in the Neonatal Context," *Theological Studies* 60 (1999).

cians, to be able to embody those values in the situations and relationships that constitute their work world. In order to enable a "lived morality," it is necessary to take into account the perceptions, motivations, and sense of identity of the person who is acting. It is here that everyday ethics and spirituality meet. [59]

This is the question of the deeper inwardness that grounds the ethical flow of relationships. In these situations, the question is added to the traditional query, What is the right thing to do? The new question probes, From what space are you doing it? In spiritual teaching, the inwardness of the acting person is crucial to the morality of the action. When actions that are meant to be caring and helpful are performed from conflicted inner spaces, they produce conflicted results. Here is an account of one caregiver's experience of the connection of spiritual inwardness and outer action.

God bless my mother, and God bless me. We made it through.

She had a stroke and a long period of rehabilitation, and it was clear she was going to have to stay with us for a while. I had all these things in mind: it was a chance to pay her back for all those years. There were these things I was going help her clear up, like the way she was thinking. I wanted to do

---

59. Cf. William C. Spohn, "Spirituality and Ethics: Exploring the Connections," *Theological Studies* (March, 1997): 109–123; Donald Evans, *Spirituality and Human Nature* (Albany, N.J.: State University of New York Press, 1993). Especially, chapters VII & VIII; Richard McCormack, *Corrective Vision: Explorations in Moral Theology* (Sheed & Ward, 1994.); Simon Harak, *Virtuous Passions: The Formation of Christian Character* (New York: Paulist, 1993); Dennis J. Billy & Donna Lynn Orsuto, *Spirituality and Morality: Integrating Prayer and Action* (New York; Paulist, 1996); Kevin T. Jackson, "Spirituality as a foundation for freedom and creative imagination in international business ethics," *Journal of Business Ethics*, 9, no. 1, (March, 1999).

the whole job very well, this big opportunity. We should all feel good about it at the end. Little things like that. Some "little!"

Fights? Classics, like only a mother and daughter can have. And my mother is a great fighter, from the Old School of somehow loving it and being very good at it and getting a kind of ecstatic look in your eye when you're really into it. I guess I'm exaggerating. It drives me a little crazy. I hate to argue. Oh, well. . . .

But it got bad. Over a hard-boiled egg we had a bad fight. We'd both gotten worn out, irritable, and frustrated. Boom! I don't remember what about—just about how it was all going and why her stay had gotten difficult and all of us had become more and more irritable and short-tempered.

In the middle of it, she stopped short and said, "Why are you doing all this for me anyway?" It sort of hit me and I started to list all the reasons. They just came out: I was afraid for her; I wanted to get her well; I felt maybe I'd ignored her when I was younger; I needed to show her I was strong; I needed to get her ready for going home alone; old age; and on and on. I was amazed myself. I could have gone on giving reasons all night. Even she was impressed.

"Junk," she said when I was done.

"Junk?" I yelled. Like, boy, she'd made a real mistake with that remark. I could really get her.

"Yes, junk," she said again, but a little more quietly. And that little-more-quietly tone got me. And she went on: "You don't have to have all those reasons. We love each other. That's enough."

I felt like a child again. Having your parents show you something that's true, but you don't feel put down—you feel better, because it is true, and you know it, even though you are a child. I said, "You're right. You're really right. I'm sorry." She said, "Don't be sorry. Junk is fine. It's what you don't need anymore. I love you."

It was a wonderful moment, and the fight stopped, which my mother accepted a little reluctantly. No, I'm joking—she was very pleased. She saw how it all was. Everything after that was just, well, easier—less pressure, less trying, less pushing, happening more by itself. And the visit ended up fine. We just spent time together, and then she went back to her house.[60]

If the intent of everyday moral actions is to change situations for the better, then the inner space of the acting person is relevant. Ethics and spirituality are partners in the development of the whole person who acts.

When the spiritual interest of ethics is characterized as a concern for the ethical problems, as a concern for the spiritual basis of ethical decision making, and as a concern for the inner state of the ethically acting person, then what spiritualities—beliefs, stories, practices—will critique and develop this interest?

Conclusion
Within a spiritually interested culture, health care becomes a spiritually interested enterprise. This interest coexists with every other organizational and medical interest. It emerges in different areas and is shaped in different ways.

---

60. Ram Dass & Paul Gorman, *How Can I Help?* (New York: Knopf, 1985), pp. 191–192.

* Patients, families, and friends are interested spiritually because it promises to provide a way to relate to losses and limits and to respond to the spiritual invitations of reconciliation, gratitude, and love that often arise within these limits and losses.

* Medical caregivers are spiritually interested in patients because it is a way to respect the whole person and to access a potential resource for physical and mental health.

* Medical caregivers are spiritually interested in themselves because it can help renew their vocational commitment and open them to enriching relationships with patients and staff.

* Chaplains are spiritually interested because it enhances their psychological and theological orientation and deepens their emphasis on self-knowledge. It also focuses their work not only on crisis moments but on overall spiritual well-being, not only on individual care but on partnership with local religious bodies, and not only on their own tradition but on the burgeoning interfaith world of patients and employees.

* The organizational life of health care is spiritually interested because it realizes that the deeper levels of employees should be recognized and included, that leaders need to be spiritually grounded to be effective in changing times, and that spiritual concern for patients and employees is a core way faith-based organizations carry out their mission.

* Ethics is spiritually interested because attempts to integrate the spiritual into various aspects of health care will precipitate ethical problems; because spiritual be-

liefs, stories, and practices enter into moral decision making; and because spiritual inwardness is an ingredient in the struggle to implement values into the everyday struggle of delivering health care.

These diverse spiritual interests constitute an openness to deeper spiritual reflection, reflection that will yield a working knowledge of the spiritual (Part Two). They also indicate a readiness to explore appropriate spiritualities, spiritualities that will allow people to pursue these interests (Part Three).

A WORKING KNOWLEDGE
OF THE SPIRITUAL

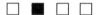

What Will Happen to the Six Spiritual Interests?

What will happen to the six spiritual interests that are emerging within health care? Will they be developed, or will they atrophy? Are they indications of future directions or, as the wag says, the "flavor of the month?"

Some think the continuation and flourishing of spiritual interests within health care depends on two factors. The first concerns the results of medical and organizational research. As medical research methods become more sophisticated, will the data continue to highlight the positive role of spirituality/religiousness in the prevention, and cure of, and coping with sickness?[1] As organizations evaluate their efforts to bring spirit into the workplace, will spirit be seen as a critical contributor to overall well-being and effectiveness? The second factor concerns the policies and programs that will implement the spiritual interest. Can spirituality be integrated into patient care in a way that is comfortable for the caregivers and not offensive to the patients? Can interfaith proselytizing, bickering, and rivalry be avoided? Can the cost of attending to patient and employee spirituality be controlled? The future of spiritual interests is closely tied to both factors—increased support from research and increased effectiveness of implementation.

Furthermore, the reality of resistance has to be considered. Although there are spiritual interests within health care, they are by no means universally welcomed. Frontline people may see the value of spirituality in their work with patients, but upper management may balk at the new organizational arrangements it would entail. Or the reverse, upper management may be eager to integrate spirituality into patient treatment for a variety of reasons, but frontline people see only more work and work for which they are not specifically trained. Integrating spirituality can be seen as an imposition, one more task in an already overworked world. By its nature, spiritual assessment and spiritual care demands time, and time is a scarce commodity in the delivery of health care. It also entails more referrals, more paperwork, more e-mails, more phone calls, and, inevitably, more failures of communications. Responding to spiritual interests may be a good

---

1. See the John L. Fetzer Institute Publication, "Multidimensional Measurement of Religiousness/Spirituality for Use in Health Research."

thing, so the argument goes, but it is one more thing. And one more thing is not needed. This is resistance that arises from the practicalities of delivering health care.

There is also theoretical resistance, and it comes from both the right and the left. Some strong faith positions see this emphasis on the spiritual as weak and watered-down. The language is vague and "vanilla." It does not reflect the richness of inherited religious language. Key ideas of religions, such as commitment, community, and tradition are not prominent. At the other end of the spectrum, humanistic perspectives do not endorse these interests. Spiritual interests are the latest examples of not respecting boundaries, of drawing outside the lines. Religion and spirituality are private matters. They belong to the intimacies of the human heart, and there are chaplains and congregations to attend to them. Why try to mainline in the medical world what is taken care of in the religious world? This is moving away from the proper calling of medicine, distracting from the real work of health care. The future of spiritual interests in health care will depend on how these practical and theoretical resistances are respected and managed.

A Working Knowledge of the Spiritual
There is still another factor influencing the future of spiritual interests in health care. It goes beyond research, implementation, and resistance, and yet, in many situations, it is not pursued. It is the great "unsaid." It concerns the fundamental vision of the spiritual, the way it is emerging, how it is being positioned in the medical and organizational landscape, and what status it is being accorded. In other words, how do we understand the spiritual that underlies the six

interests and is the provisional basis for welcoming and developing spiritualities? What is needed is a working knowledge of the spiritual, a knowledge that gives us some of the key features of the reality we are talking about. A working knowledge is more than a commonly agreed upon definition, but it does not strive for complete comprehension or consider its subject in the abstract. Rather, it entails a familiarity with the subject in the specific context in which it is being considered. When people within health care are interested in the spiritual, what might the spiritual in which they are interested look like?

Although the spiritual has never been absent from health care, it is now being envisioned and included in a different way. The recognition of the spiritual as an essential dimension of the human is the foundation of this new way. The spiritual is "there," a given of human existence and a "player" in all experiences of health and sickness. The only options are to include it or ignore it. But whether it is included or ignored, it is still "there." And, as H.L. Mencken once said about the essential mysteriousness of life, no matter how much it is ignored, it sits there "calmly licking its chops."[2]

This "givenness" of the spiritual means that it includes, but goes beyond, organized religion. Taking it into account is more than a religious preference or even a religious obligation. It is a fundamental human responsibility. That understanding is reflected in the instructions of the Joint Commission on Accreditation of Health Care Organizations.

---

2. Quoted in Larry Dossey, *Healing Words* (San Francisco: HarperSanFrancisco, 1993) p. 80.

The purpose of a spiritual assessment is to evaluate such factors as the client's relationship with humanity and with God or a higher power. It might include the client's philosophical orientation toward the purpose and meaning of life. It is not intended to be confined solely to identifying the client's religion. Says Hansen, "Knowing an individual's spiritual, cultural, and social value system is the key ingredient to understanding the individual's perception of treatment outcome and continued stability."[3]

The spiritual is a dimension that has to be taken into account if health care is to treat individuals in their concrete particularities.

If this new positioning and status of the spiritual is fully understood and accepted, it legitimates the pursuit and development of spiritual interests. Research will continue to uncover new connections and nuance and interrelate the data, implementation will remain a challenge and progress in its usual trial-and-error fashion, resistance and compliance will always be a matter of shifting percentages. However, none of these changing conditions will invalidate the inclusion of the spiritual.

Therefore, it is important to grasp this new status and positioning of the spiritual. Of course, to people on the spirituality side of the conversation this sounds strange. The spiritual is not a new situation but a primordial condition. It is not only essential to the human, it is the ultimate core of the human. The most profound truth about humanity is its combination of relatedness and estrangement from the Divine

---

3. Joint Commission Perspectives (July/August 1999): 15.

Spirit. However, it is not the spiritual "per se" that is under consideration. It is how the spiritual is appreciated, how it is acknowledged, how it is included. Spiritual sensitivity is an always present companion of the human, but it is being introduced in a new way. It is this reintroduction that grounds, legitimates, and shapes the emerging spiritual interests. In short, what is needed is a working knowledge of the spiritual.

The New Kid on the Medical Block

In *Kitchen Table Wisdom,* Rachel Remen recounts her teenage experience as a volunteer in a nursing home for the aged.[4] She was given the task of trying to engage a ninety-six-year-old woman in conversation. The woman had been diagnosed as having senile dementia and had not talked to anyone in more than a year. The nursing staff did not think the woman would talk to Rachel, so they gave her a basket of glass beads. The plan was that she and the woman would string beads together.

When Rachel arrived at the room, the woman was sitting in a chair facing a window. The morning light was pouring in. There was another chair facing the window. Rachel sat down. She tried to think of some way to engage the woman, but nothing seemed like it would work. Finally, she just gave up and sat for the full hour with the basket of glass beads on her lap.

When she was leaving, curiosity overcame her. She asked the woman what she was looking at. "Slowly she turned to-

---

4. Rachel Naomi Remen, M.D., *Kitchen Table Wisdom* (New York: Riverhead Books, 1994) pp. 23–25.

ward me and I could see her face for the first time. It was radiant. In a voice filled with joy she said, "Why, child, I am looking at the Light."

Remen reflects: "A ninety-six-year-old woman may stop speaking because arteriosclerosis has damaged her brain, or she has become psychotic and she is no longer able to speak. But she may also have withdrawn into a space between the worlds, to contemplate what is next, to spread her sails and patiently wait to catch the light."

This progression of possible explanations for the woman not talking reflects the contemporary way the spiritual is approached. First, the physical influence on her condition is acknowledged (arteriosclerosis); then the psychological is entertained (psychotic); finally, the spiritual is brought forward (a space between worlds). The spiritual is considered as one more "take" on the situation. The spiritual perspective is not necessarily in competition with the physical and the psychological observations. They can all reflect a piece of the actual situation. However, the spiritual is brought in last, as a suggestive and complementary "maybe."

This "newness" of the spiritual is reflected in another physician's firsthand account. Dr. Arthur Kornhaber was researching the relationship between grandparents and grandchildren when he noticed "things taking place that could not be adequately explained by psychological theory."[5] For example, one day he brought some elementary schoolchildren into a nursing home. One girl, Annie, who was around seven years old, spotted an old woman alone by herself. She was

---

5. Arthur Kornhaber, M.D., *Spirit: Mind, Body, and the Will to Existence* (New York: St. Martin's Press, 1988) p. 12.

sitting in a wheelchair, a belt tied around her waist keeping her upright. Her clothes were disheveled. Overall, she was lifeless. Annie approached her and told her she liked her dress. Kornhaber wandered away to check on the other children. When he returned, Annie and the old woman could not be found. The nurse told him Annie had wheeled Mrs. Boyce back to her room. "It's room 112."

When Dr. Kornhaber entered the room, he couldn't believe his eyes. Mrs. Boyce was transformed. She was sitting up straight, her eyes were bright and there was life in her movements. She was combing Annie's hair, and the two of them were chatting away. Annie turned to Kornhaber and said excitedly, "She knew my grandpa!"

The medical researcher in Kornhaber immediately goes to work.

What I now call my half-mind went to work on it. Reflex medical, psychological thoughts raced through my brain, frantically trying to give "reason" to this occurrence. Did Annie remind Mrs. Boyce of someone or something in her past that activated her memory? Was it just that Annie's presence simply engaged Mrs. Boyce's interest because usually she had no such stimulation? And then did these phenomena cause her body to react by pumping adrenaline into her bloodstream, which would explain her "activation"?

Although these explanations were plausible, they didn't "feel" right, they were not sufficient, in my view, to explain the extent of Mrs. Boyce's sudden and unexplained vitality. So it came to mind that perhaps Mrs. Boyce wasn't revitalized because her thyroid or adrenal glands pumped hormones into her bloodstream, but that the opposite was true: Her

glands were pumping because she was vitalized—spirited—
by some close interaction with the little girl. At this point I
stopped myself short. "Wait a minute," I said to myself. "This
idea is off the wall."

Once again the spiritual comes in last, and it is considered
in its interactions with the more established knowledge of the
physical and social-psychological dimensions.

A third example of "bringing in" the spiritual is Harold
Koenig's description of a more complete approach to health
and aging. He notes that physical, psychological, and social
perspectives are not enough to account for what is happening.

"The biopsychosocial model, which operates on a systems
approach, seeks to integrate all aspects of the human being
and his or her world: the biological, psychological, and interpersonal. Because of the overriding importance of religion
in the lives of so many older Americans and the needs that it
fulfills, the biopsychosocial model cannot exclude the spiritual and still be called complete; thus, the need arises for a
biopsychosocial-spiritual model of health and aging." [6]

This text clearly states the company into which the spiritual
is invited. The spiritual is introduced as a complementary
dimension to approaches that are already well-established in
the field of health care. The biological, psychological, and
interpersonal (social) have previously covered the territory.

---

6. Harold G. Koenig, "Religion and Health in Later Life," in *Aging, Spirituality, and Religion: A Handbook*. (Minneapolis: Fortress, 1995).

There is a vast amount of research and theory about how these dimensions work and how they influence one another. Now, in the name of completeness, the spiritual needs to be added. The spiritual enters the line-up as one more perspective to take into account. Koenig suggests it is added more by popular demand than scientific necessity. It is what the aging people themselves consider important.

A fourth example of the inclusion of the spiritual can be seen in a 1997 report the Institute for the Future presented to The Robert Wood Johnson Foundation. It is a preliminary forecast entitled "Piecing Together the Puzzle: The Future of Health and Health Care in America." The report includes a section on an expanded perspective on health and disease. It envisions going beyond a narrowly conceived biomedical model of health and disease to consider four contributors and determinants of health—physical, mental, social, and spiritual. However, in response to a section entited "What's New," the report states, "Dependence on a biomedical model to define disease and health has been rendered insufficient by a growing body of evidence that health involves much more than freedom from active disease or illness, and that up-stream environmental and psychosocial determinants of disease deserve parity with conventional biological theories." Although the spiritual is included as part of the new situation of health care earlier in the report, in this section it is not explicitly mentioned. I suspect the reason for its omission is that it is the latest member of the team. It is acknowledged, but, at the present time, not deeply understood or integrated with other approaches. The spiritual is the "new kid on the block." It is being invited into a medial and organizational world strongly defined by physical, psychological, and social networks.

A Dimensional Model of Health Care

These four aspects of the human—physical, psychological, social, and spiritual—can be considered as interlocking dimensions. Each has its own distinctiveness and yet each is capable of influencing the others. Together they form a dimensional model that is increasingly used in health care settings. Models are maps to the territory, not the territory itself. They are used to the extent they make the terrain visible, especially terrain that formerly had gone unnoticed. They are discarded when more adequate maps are drawn. This dimensional model has considerable mapping ability. It focuses on the four dimensions as always present, as mutually influential, and as distinctive in their own right.[7]

First, the four dimensions are present in every experience. Although in health care, the physical and psychological dimensions are usually prominent, the social and spiritual dimensions are also present. This firsthand account of an office visit shows how all the dimensions are present and embedded in one another.

I sat in the specialist's office. He came in with a large white envelope that I knew carried films of my back and head. He

---

7. For an appreciation of a dimensional approach from a theological perspective, see Paul Tillich, *Systematic Theology*, vol. III (Chicago: University of Chicago Press, 1963); Jerry Gill, *On Knowing God* (Philadelphia: Westminster Press, 1981); John Cobb, *Theology and Pastoral Care* (Minneapolis: Fortress, 1977).

sat down and without any emotion he simply said, "You have MS."

I had expected it. My family doctor had given me the same diagnosis. But I had insisted on seeing a specialist. All my friends urged me on.

"Are you sure?" I asked. I guess I was in denial.

"I would bet my practice on it, " he said.

I was on the seventeenth floor of a plush office building on Michigan Ave. This man was not a reckless gambler with his practice. I guess I had ms.

I looked over at my husband who was sitting next to me. He was crying. For the first time I realized this was not my disease alone. My husband and family were in it with me. Everyone was affected.

"God help us," I said inside myself where no one could hear it.

Her physical situation (multiple sclerosis) initiates the whole process. She guesses she is in denial (psychological), notices and realizes her husband's involvement (social), and spontaneously and interiorly reaches for divine help (spiritual). Although any given experience may be initiated in one dimension, it always includes the total person, touching, sooner or later, on every dimension.[8]

The presence of every dimension in every experience is the grounding for some crucial distinctions in health care. Dis-

---

8. "Restoration of the patient's health requires elimination of the disease if that is possible, but in addition it requires that attention be directed to the patient's mental, social and spiritual well-being in keeping with an expanded view of health." "Piecing Together the Puzzle: The Future of Health and Health Care in America," The Institute for the Future.

ease is often distinguished from illness. Disease is the physiological process, and illness is the social experience of that process.[9] Curing and healing are also distinguished. Curing focuses on the cessation of the physical disease or impairment. Healing focuses on the psychological wholeness, social reconciliation, or spiritual communion that has occurred during the course of the disease. Healing and curing can coexist, but healing can happen when there is no cure. Finally, pain and suffering are distinguished. Once again, pain points to the physiological trauma that is occurring, and suffering looks to the total human response to that trauma. Psychological, social, and spiritual factors can exasperate the pain and heighten the total suffering or be supportive in such a way that the total suffering is reduced. These distinctions show that the same experience can be looked at from physical, psychological, social, and spiritual points of view. The result is diverse appreciations of what is possible in the experience of sickness.

When these dimensions are not taken into account in health care settings, there is a danger of reducing a person to their physical status. In Margaret Edson's Pulitzer prize-winning play, *Wit*, Vivian Bearing, the main character, reflects that her doctors will probably write an article about her.

But I flatter myself. The article will not be about *me*, it will be about my ovaries. It will be about my peritoneal cavity,

9. For the danger of turning this distinction into a separation, see Arthur W. Frank, *The Wounded Storyteller* (Chicago: The University of Chicago Press, 1995).

which, despite their best intentions, is now crawling with cancer.

What we have come to think of as me is, in fact, just the specimen jar, the dust jacket, just the white piece of paper that bears the little black marks.[10]

When a dimensional understanding of the human person does not direct our health care efforts, we become whatever is happening to our bodies. This reduction is the chronic temptation of the biomedical approach.

Second, these dimensions are mutually influential. Of course, the predominant medical interest is how the psychological, social, and spiritual dimensions influence the physical. Since medicine is primarily interested in physical well-being, it interrogates the other dimensions from that point of view. However, influences run in all directions. Disturbances in the physical dimension have precipitated spiritual evaluation and change.[11] Spiritual experience has been the driving force behind social change.[12] Psychological counseling has been a path to both physical relief and social reconciliation. The dimensions interact in diverse and often baffling ways.

---

10. Margaret Edson, *Wit* (Winchester, Mass.: Faber and Faber, 1999), p. 53.
11. See Mary Farrell Bednarowski, "Theological Creativity: Personalizing Religious Traditions Can Help The Healing Process," *The Park Ridge Center Bulletin* (January-February 1999).
12. The Biblical traditions, in particular the prophetic strand, have held together the spiritual and the social. A correct relationship to the Divine Source has always included a realignment of social structures. The Ten Commandments embody this connection. The first tablet constructs the relationship to God; the second tablet spells out the implications for the relationship to neighbor. Neither tablet stands alone; each needs the other.

The fact that the dimensions influence one another is commonly accepted. But the degree to which they can influence one another, the exact way the influence occurs, and whether or not the influence can be predicted is highly debated. Therefore, what needs to be explored are the paths and connections between the dimensions. For example, in Buddhist teaching, insight into the spiritual truth of impermanence unfolds into the social virtue of compassion. But what are the steps, the interior logic, the sequence of perceptions, and stirrings of will that move impermanence into compassion? Another example concerns the research on meditation. Meditation quiets the mind and, in turn, has the effect of lowering blood pressure. But how exactly does this happen, and what happens when meditation is over? Is consciousness the pathway between the mental and physical dimensions? One benefit of the dimensional model is it allows us both to see influences and encourages us to explore the path of influence.[13]

Third, each dimension has its distinctive laws and operations, and so no dimension can substitute for another. The dimensions are mutually influential, but they are not reducible to each other. The laws and operations of physical reality are not the same as the laws and operations of spiritual reality, and how the psyche works is not the same as how

---

13. "That spiritual factors promote good health; aid in the recovery from illness, and contribute to the state of well-being that characterizes health has growing support. The questions are how and why? The mental, social and spiritual components of health may have distinctive but similar salutary effect mediated through psychoneuroendocrine pathways." "Piecing Together the Puzzle: The Future of Health and Health Care in America," The Institute for the Future.

society works. Each dimension has its own integrity and should be respected on its own terms. This is often difficult to do, and there has been a long history of one dimension infringing on another and one dimension being reduced to another.[14]

At one point in human awareness, the events of each dimension—the physical, the psychological, the social, and the spiritual—were interpreted from a spiritual perspective. The response to infertility was prayer, the response to mental illness was exorcism, defeat in battle could be traced to the sinfulness of people. The spiritual dimension was monolithic, exercising control in every other dimension. On the surface, it may have appeared that the dimensions were unified within the embrace of the supreme dimension, the spiritual. But on closer inspection and from the vantage point of hindsight, what was present was an undifferentiated mass. The spiritual was infringing on all the other dimensions.

This situation changed dramatically. People began to see that the physical, psychological, and social dimensions had an integrity of their own. The events of these dimensions could be interpreted on their own terms. Infertility could be worked with physiologically, mental illness could be negotiated with drugs and counseling, the immediate causes of war were economic and political. The spiritual was, sometimes quietly but most of the time vociferously, pushed out. It now had little or no interpretive power in the other dimensions.

---

14. For an insightful and extensive unfolding of this history, see Ken Wilber, *Eye to Eye: The Quest for a New Paradigm* (Boston: Shambhala, 1990). Also, Langdon Gilkey, *Religion in a Scientific Future* (New York: Harper & Row, 1979); and Langdon Gilkey, "The New Watershed in Theology," *Soundings* (Summer, 1981).

The dethroning of the spiritual did not stop there, however. The exponents of the physical, psychological, and social dimensions trained their "way of doing things" on specifically spiritual experience. In their estimation, they could account for the religious data in a more persuasive way than religion and spirituality could. Theologians quickly labeled this effort reductionism[15]: the spiritual dimension of life was reduced to the physical, psychological, or social. This intrusion into the spiritual domain could be looked at as the other dimensions returning the favor. The spiritual had interpreted their proper domain. Now they were interpreting the proper domain of the spiritual. The result of this development—the exclusion of the spiritual from the physical, psychological, and social and the consequent interpretation of the spiritual by the physical, psychological, and social—was secularism. Secular consciousness simply excluded the spiritual from its way of perceiving reality.

The advent of secular consciousness momentarily took the spiritual out of contention. Although this truncated the fullness of the human condition, it gave the physical, psychological, and social dimensions time and energy to explore their specific domains. The result was that they established themselves firmly in human awareness. There may be many theo-

---

15. Theologians gave it a name, but the novelist John Updike caught the feeling. One of his characters rambles: "Whenever theology touches science it get burned. In the sixteenth century astronomy, in the seventeenth microbiology, in the eighteenth geology and paleontology, in the nineteenth Darwin's biology, all grotesquely extended the world-frame and sent churchmen scurrying for cover in ever smaller shadowy nooks, little gloomy ambiguous caves in the psyche where even now neurology is cruelly harrying them, gouging them out from the multifolded brain like wood lice from under the lumber pile." *Roger's Version* (New York: Knopf, 1986).

ries and practices associated with the physical dimension of existence, but the physical itself is a field of inquiry with appropriate boundaries and procedures. The same is true of the other two dimensions. The psychological and social are approached in a multitude of ways, but in themselves they are established fields of inquiry, essential aspects of the human. Once this line-up was established and confident, it invited the spiritual back in. But the rules of the game had changed.

As a result, the spiritual is not being introduced in either of its past roles. It is not portrayed as the dominant player that controls the other dimensions or as a mere epiphenomenon, reducible to physical, psychological, or social dynamics. The excesses that made the spiritual everything or nothing are avoided. It is now seen as a complementary dimension with its own laws, operations, and modes of knowing. It is an acknowledged component of a new model of differentiated unity, a model that maps human experience as dimensional and the dimensions as both interactive and distinctive.

Implications for Religious Traditions

When the spiritual is viewed as a dimension of human experience interacting with other dimensions yet having its own distinctiveness, there are a number of implications for religious traditions.

First, the spiritual is not exclusively identified with organized religious traditions.[16] People become aware of the spiri-

---

16. For a strong case that religion is only one path among many to the spiritual, see David N. Elkins, *Beyond Religion* (Wheaton, Il: Theosophical Publishing House, 1998). For a sharp distinction between spirituality and religion, a distinction to the point of separation, see Beatrice Bruteau, "Cre-

tual in a variety of settings—a mother nursing a baby, two friends conversing, a man gazing at the night stars, a woman wholeheartedly serving another person, a child playing in the grass. The spiritual is an always present dimension of life, and so it can break into consciousness at any time. In a recent study, physicians asked about their spirituality recounted experiences they had with patients, times when there was a spiritual quality about the interaction. They did not volunteer moments of prayer or religious ritual. Their natural inclination was to search the world of their everyday experience. It seems many people become conscious of the spiritual in nonreligious settings and so are capable of saying, "I'm

---

ative Spirituality: Knowing By Being." *The Quest* (Summer, 1998) p. 17. She writes, "Spirituality is always outside the churches—or temples or mosques. Spirituality is something different from religion. Spirituality transcends creeds, cults and codes of behavior. Religion concerns itself with giving meaning to life for a community of believers; it is, to a great extent, stylized and shared in common. It has boundaries set by sacred scriptures, traditions, holy places and people, authoritative institutions. You can define the rules for belonging to a given religion, and that religion in turn will help to define you. You can say that you are a Presbyterian or a Vaishnavite or a Theravadin or a Shite or a Hasid, and console yourself that you know a little better who you are and where you fit into the world and even into the Reality beyond the world.

Spirituality isn't like that. It doesn't offer any preformed set of answers to chosen questions, or an obligatory way of life, or a community in which to share such beliefs and behaviors and thus feel at home, confident that you are right. Spirituality means a quest, a personal quest for reality and truth— whatever they turn out to be. There isn't any revealed spirituality or any heretical spirituality; no inerrant or infallible or guaranteed spirituality. Spirituality isn't a comfort, it's a risk. It has no given style, you have to create it as you go along. It has no boundaries, but continues to be open, unfinished. You can't define it, and it can't define you. On the contrary, to be on a spiritual quest means that you question and may forsake all your familiar definitions."

probably not very religious, but I consider myself a deeply spiritual person."[17]

This emphasis on the universal presence of the spiritual lights up the contemporary landscape in a complex way. Some people can be spiritual without belonging to an organized religious tradition. Some people who belong to an organized religious tradition may not participate in that tradition in a spiritual way, and so they can be religious without being spiritual. For other people, their membership and participation in an organized religious tradition is a genuine spiritual path, and so they are both religious and spiritual.[18] Also, people can be encouraged to bring spirit into work settings, a spirit that is seen as stimulating excellence and cooperation. In the same breath, however, faith and religion are discouraged.[19] They may be seen as both irrelevant and contributing to disagreements and tensions. Furthermore, patients may report that a hospital with no religious affiliation is a spiritually vibrant facility while a religiously sponsored hospital is a cold and unwelcoming place. Once the spiritual is conceived as a dimension of the human and, therefore, capable of "bubbling up" anywhere, different ways of looking at and evaluating religion and the spiritual come into being.

17. See Meredith B. McGuire, "Mapping Contemporary American Spirituality: A Sociological Perspective," *Christian Spirituality Bulletin* (Spring, 1997) pp. 1–8.

18. For a nuanced way of understanding the co-occurence of religion and spirituality, see David B. Larson, James P. Sawyers, and Michael E. McCullough, *Scientific Research on Spirituality and Health: A Consensus Report* (National Institute for Health Care Research,1998).

19. See Ian I. Mitroff and Elizabeth A. Denton, *A Spiritual Audit of Corporate America: A Hard Look at Spirituality, Religion and Values in the Workplace* (San Francisco: Jossey-Bass Publishers, 1999).

Second, this distinction between the spiritual and religious traditions pressures religions to reclaim their spiritual identity. Religious traditions are the primary home of the spiritual. They are founded on revelations of the spiritual and carry the majority of the spiritual wisdom of the human race. Even when people wake up to the spiritual through experiences that are not facilitated by the beliefs and rituals of a religious tradition, they usually search out the significance of those experiences by consulting some representatives of religious traditions. Also, intensive and prolonged training in the spiritual life is carried on within religious traditions and communities. Thus, religious traditions are the context of and provide support for individual spiritual seeking. In the best scenario, personal spiritual experience and religious traditions are partners in the spiritual development of people.

This partnership encourages religious traditions to retrieve and bring forward their treasures. It is not enough just to cite past teachings and pioneering people who embodied a spiritually passionate life in the religious and social swirl of their times. Any historical appreciation has to be joined to the distinctive contemporary struggles of spiritual living. There must be an imaginative "bringing forward," a connecting of past spiritual wisdom and contemporary situations. For example, if features of the Christian spiritual tradition of *ars moriendi* (the art of dying) are to be brought forward, they must relate to the medical and social realities of dying in today's society. If spiritual exercises that encourage "contemplation in action" are offered, it must be remembered that they are offered to people in the heat and harry of urban life. This is a challenging time for religious traditions. They are being called upon to remember the deepest truth about themselves—their spiritual identity—and to present that truth as a gift to seeking people.

Third, the emphasis on the spiritual as a universal dimension provides a way to appreciate the ecumenical (the varying denominations within Christianity) and interfaith environment of contemporary health care. American culture is increasingly an ecumenical and interfaith reality, and health care reflects this pluralism in both its employees and its patients. How will this religiously plural situation be understood and played out? A first level advocates mere tolerance. Pluralism is the situation, and it is here to stay. Even if you do not like it, you have to learn to live with it. A second level distinguishes faith motivation and grounding from practical, concrete issues. It suggests bracketing the faith material and cooperating as much as possible in practical matters. No matter what the faith backdrop, everyone can work for excellence in medical treatment and greater patient satisfaction. Once the spiritual is recognized as an essential element, however, there is a call to go beyond tolerance and practicality.

The next step is respect and dialogue. The many faith traditions are respected because they are expressions of the spiritual possibilities of the human. They witness to how this important level of life is symbolized and courted by people seeking the fullness of human development. A part of this respect is that the people or organizations of one faith tradition (e.g., Christian) encourage the people or organizations of another faith tradition (e.g., Jewish) to reach into their own tradition for the spiritual resources that are available.[20]

---

20. Advocate Health Care has formulated a statement about the interfaith nature of health care—*Advocate as Faith-Based: A Renewed Focus.*

This depth of respect leads to dialogue in which people begin to understand the heart of their own faith and how it can be complemented and resourced by the heart of another faith. All dialogue is a wager, and interfaith dialogue is often a difficult conversation. But it is a conversation made necessary by a socially plural world and the recognition of the spiritual as essential to human well-being.

Attending to the Spiritual

Herbert Benson has characterized health care as a three-legged stool—pharmaceuticals, surgery, and self-care.[21] The emphasis on self-care is a recent addition, and it fits in well with the overall cultural value on leading an intentional life.[22] People are encouraged to become responsible for their health by engaging in activities that will promote it and avoiding

---

"Advocate respects and encourages the specific faiths of all peoples, both patients and associates.

In interviews with Advocate leadership, it was consistently stressed that the faith-based nature of Advocate must strive to be inclusive. In the past, stressing a specific religious faith often led, on the one hand, to proselytizing and, on the other hand, to acrimony and division. The solution seemed to be to avoid the question of faith. This screened out an important aspect of people's commitment and motivation, even though, on the surface, it seemed to promote harmony. If you wanted to live side by side in a pluralistic society, the path of advancement seemed to be to become "faith-blind." Faith was an individual choice and a private matter.

Advocate seeks a different way. It acknowledges, respects, and encourages the diverse faiths of individuals in our pluralistic society. This respect is engendered by Advocate's Christian heritage. As a Christian faith-based organization, it recognizes faith as a universal human reality and welcomes people of all faiths along the path of health and healing. This is a journey together that will take place step by step. Whatever arises—whether differences or convergences—will be met in a spirit of respect and openness."

21. Herbert Benson, "The Faith-Factor: An Interview with Herbert Benson," *Common Boundary* (July/August 1997).

22. See Paul N. Duckro, "An Intentional Life," *Church* (Spring 1994) pp. 14–17.

activities that will endanger it. The overly optimistic admonition is, "Take care of yourself now, so others do not have to take of you later." This stress on self-care does not mean no one else is involved, but it does single out the individual as a proactive pusurer of health and the ultimate bearer of responsibility. This is a far cry from being the passive patient whose sole role in the pursuit of health was compliance with the doctor's orders. Rather, people are encouraged to lead an intentional life, aware of the complexities involved in maintaining health and attentive to their overall well-being.

If we understand ourselves according to the dimensional model, the agenda of self-care unfolds logically. We attend to the health of our body, paying attention to diet and exercise. In order to do this, we may consult a dietitian, read books on healthy and unhealthy foods, learn stretching and strengthening exercises from a physical therapist, and so forth. We also will go to doctors for check-ups and undergo procedures to determine whether there are any hidden causes of disease. In other words, we attend to the health of our bodies by connecting with key other people and becoming consumers of knowledges and services that will help us.

We also attend to the health of our psyche. Often this entails a wide variety of activities. It may include intellectual and artistic stimulation—learning new things, attending classes, keeping abreast of change. We may discover that darker regions of the psyche need to be explored, and so we see a counselor or therapist to become more aware of what drives us. We also are careful not to overtax ourselves with too many people or too much work. In the process of attending to our psychological health, we come to a realistic personal assessment of our limits and our reach.

We also attend to our social health in its many aspects. We look for meaningful work in a humane environment with the best compensation we can find. We change employers until we come to the best situation. We nurture our relationships with family and friends. We try to give priority to our personal lives and not take whatever love is in our lives for granted. In order to do this, we probably have to make continual adjustments, especially with regard to how we use our time. Time is the opportunity to love. We fear we will squander it on less important things. This social aspect of ourselves is essentially interpersonal, and so the responsibility for cultivating relationships is communally shared by family, friends, coworkers, neighbors, and even fellow citizens.

The logical next step would be to develop at length ways in which we care for ourselves spiritually. Although this language of "caring for the spiritual" or "caring for the soul" is both rooted in certain religious traditions and currently popular, it may be misleading. It might obscure the distinctiveness of the spiritual. Although the spiritual influences the physical, psychological, and social, its laws and operations are decidedly different. It is peculiar and its ways are often advertised as unconventional, and strange.[23] In the Hebrew scriptures, this difference is placed in the mouth of God. "For my thoughts are not your thoughts, nor are your ways my ways, says the Lord. For as the heavens are higher than the earth, so are my ways higher than your ways, my thoughts higher than your thoughts" (Isaiah 55:8–9). Flannery O'Connor was fond of saying about spiritual truth, "You will

---

23. See John Shea, *Starlight* (New York: Crossroad, 1992), pp. 47–74.

know the truth and the truth will make you odd."[24] Theologian David Tracy uses the phrase "uncanny" to emphasize the advent of spiritual reality.[25] We need to explore the peculiarity, oddness, and uncanniness of the spiritual and its ways before we develop advice on how to attend to it. However, since our task is to sketch a working knowledge of the spiritual, we will focus on only a few of its salient features. In particular, we will explore how the awareness of the spiritual is an inner path that opens the two eyes of the soul and receives Spirit as a resource for the struggles of living.

An Inner Path

Although the spiritual dimension is always present, people are not aware of it. If we think of this in terms of images, we can say we have a vintage wine cellar, and we rarely drink from it. We have an interior castle, and we seldom visit it. There is a treasure buried in our field, and we do not know how to unearth it. The first line of Denise Levertov's poem "Flickering Mind" expresses this as "Lord, not you / it is I who am absent."[26] Thomas Merton said, "We are living in a world that is absolutely transparent and God is shining through it all the time. . . . The only thing is we don't see it." [27] Therefore, the distinction between the presence of the spiritual and the awareness of the spiritual is foundational in spiritual teach-

---

24. Quoted in Harry Moody, *The Five Stages of the Soul* (New York: Doubleday, 1997).

25. David Tracy, *The Analogical Imagination* (New York: Crossroad, 1981).

26. Denise Levertov, *The Stream and the Sapphire* (New York: New Dimensions Books, 1997), p. 15.

27. Quoted in Marcus J. Borg, *The God We Never Knew* (San Francisco: HarperSanFrancisco, 1997).

ing and sets in motion the spiritual project. We are asleep, and we need to awake; we are blind, and we need to see; we are deaf, and we need to hear; we are lost, and we need to be found; we are dead, and we need to come back to life. All these images point to the spiritual venture of becoming aware of what is there.[28]

Often we are not aware of the spiritual because we are looking in the wrong direction. Our consciousness is always outside ourselves. The five senses pull awareness into the outer world, a world of enticements that is constantly soliciting our attention. Spiritual teaching, on the other hand, suggests we reverse the process and pull consciousness inside. It follows the insight of Augustine, "I was outside. You were within." In Hindu literature this interior move is called "the turtle pulls in its feet." That is what it feels like, a movement toward inner exploration. However, it is important to note that the spiritual is not inside as opposed to outside. Rather "going inside" is how we become aware of the spiritual that is both within and without. In order to discern the spiritual dimension of everything, we first have to know it as the ground of our own being.[29]

---

28. For approaches to the spiritual that emphasize consciousness, see, among others, Willis W. Harmon and Christian De Quincy, *The Scientific Exploration of Consciousness: Toward an Adequate Epistemology* (Institute of Noetic Sciences, 1994); Ramakrishna Puligandla, *An Encounter with Awareness* (Wheaton, Il: Theosophical Publishing House, 1981); Beatrice Bruteau, *The Psychic Grid: How We Create the World We Know* (Wheaton, Il.: The Theosophical Publishing House, 1979); Stanislav Grof, ed., *Human Survival and Consciousness Evolution*, (Albany: State University of New York Press, 1988).

29. "God cannot be found or grasped in the external world, but only in the inner world. If we seek him outside, we shall find him nowhere; if we seek him within, we shall find him everywhere. This is not to say that only the

This inner path is essential to attending to the spiritual. The Jesus of the Gospel of Thomas goes beyond the Jesus of the Gospel of Luke who merely says, "The Kingdom is within you."

> If those who lead you say to you,
> 'See, the kingdom is in the sky'
> then the birds of the sky will precede you.
>
> If they say to you,
> 'It is in the sea,'
> then the fish of the sea will precede you.
>
> If you will know yourselves,
> then you will be known and you will know
> that you are sons and daughters of the Living One.
>
> But if you do not know yourselves,
> then you are in poverty and you are poverty. (Gospel of Thomas, 3)

This text connects the Kingdom within with knowing yourself. "Know thyself" is a foundational maxim of the spiritual life. Plotinus elaborated on this directive writing, "we must close our eyes and invoke a new manner of seeing, a wake-

---

inner world is real. Both are real; both have their own measure of importance. But it is the inner world which has the priority and the greater importance. . . . Having discovered God within, we can discover him without; but never the other way round." Cyprian Smith, *The Way of Paradox* (New York: Paulist Press, 1987), p. 51.

fulness that is the birthright of us all, though few put it to use." The closed eyes take us away from the outer world into an inner landscape we see in a new way, where a sighting of the spiritual dimension is possible. Once consciousness is pulled out of the social swirl, it goes within and encounters the body and mind. In other words, it attends to the physical and mental dimensions of the human person.[30] However, this is only the beginning of the inner journey. There comes a moment when we realize we are always more than what we are seeing. This is the discovery of what theology calls the transcendent self. It is not a datum of consciousness so much as it is coinciding with consciousness itself.[31] Ken Wilber elaborates on this realization:

> You needn't try to see your transcendent self, which is not possible anyway. Can your eye see itself? You need only begin by persistently dropping your false identifications with your memories, mind, body, emotions, and thoughts. And this dropping entails nothing by way of super-human effort or theoretical comprehension. All that is required, primarily, is but one understanding: whatever you can see cannot be the Seer. Everything you know about yourself is precisely not your Self, the Knower, the inner I-ness that can neither be perceived, defined, or made an object of any sort. Bondage is nothing but the mis-identification of the Seer with all these

---

30. For a developed account of this interior process, see John Shea, *Gospel Light: Jesus Stories for Spiritual Consciousnes* (New York: Crossroad, 1998), chap. 1: "The Way of Spiritual Consciousness."
31. For the importance of this distinction, see Gerald May, *Simply Sane* (New York: Crossroad, 1993), p. 80.

things which can be seen. And liberation begins with the simple reversal of this mistake.[32]

This realization of consciousness goes by many names. Besides the transcendent self, it is called the deep self, the real self, the ultimate self, essence, and the true self. These names signify how valuable it is to discover this treasure, this forgotten pearl.[33]

The Two Eyes of the Soul

In traditional religious imagery, this inner space of awareness is also called the soul. Following the Arab philosopher Avicenna, many Western spiritual teachers imagined the soul as having two eyes.[34] One eye peered into the eternal, and one eye peered into the temporal.[35] This made the spiritual identity of the human person a boundary reality, joining spirit and flesh, heaven and earth, the eternal and the temporal. In ancient categories, humans are neither angels (pure spirits) nor animals (pure matter). They are the intermingling and flow of spirit and matter.

Therefore, on the one hand, the soul is the primordial

---

32. Ken Wilber, *No Boundary* (Boston: Shambhala Press, 1979), p. 137.

33. See the Gnostic story, "The Hymn of the Pearl." It is recalled and interpreted in Harry Moody, *The Five Stages of the Soul* (New York: Doubleday, 1997).

34. See *The Theological Germanica of Martin Luther*, trans. Bengt Hoffman (New York: Paulist Press, 1980). p. 64. "The created soul of man has two eyes. One (the right) represents the power to peer into the eternal. The other (the left) gazes into time and the created world."

35. For an interesting assesment tool that holds together "both eyes," that relates people's relationship to God with their psychological sense of well-being, see Jared Kass, "Tapping Into Something Greater Than Ourselves," *Spirituality and Health* (Fall 1996).

connectedness of the human person with the Sacred, or Spirit, or God (or with whatever other words denote Ultimate Reality). On the other hand, soul points to the connection of the human person with the mind-body organism and through that organism with the entire world. Soul is both the "organ of communion" with God and the form that energizes and is present in every aspect of the mind-body.[36] To emphasize this inclusive and connective power, Georges Poulet stresses that the soul should be considered a center: "It is a center, not only, as the mystics believe, because God has in it His chosen abode, but because this place of divine dwelling is also the convergence of all cosmic phenomena."[37] It is this inclusiveness and centrality of soul that encourages people when they are in soul consciousness to say simply, "I am." They sense they are defined by a communion with existence itself and with all that participates in existence. This is who they are.[38]

Understanding the two eyes of the soul is important for discussions about spirituality in health care. Many characterize spirituality as supplying a transcendent perspective or giving meaning and purpose to the events of life and to life in general. In other words, they are focusing on the eye of

---

36. "The essence of the soul . . . and that which constitutes its worth, is its being the organ of communion with God." Remi Brague, "The Soul of Salvation," *Communio* (Fall 1987) p: 226.

37. Quoted in Thomas Keating, M. Basil Pennington, and Thomas E. Clarke, *Finding Grace at the Center* (Still River, Mass.: St. Bede Publications, 1978).

38. Cf. this first hand account from David Brandon "Nowness in the Helping Relationship," in *Awakening The Heart* ed. by John Weldwood (New Science Library, 1985). "Outside the wintry afternoon gave way to darkness and a biting wind. I walked up and down in a very large, high-ceilinged stable. My stride quickened and I kicked out pieces of stick and stones. The ques-

the soul that peers into the temporal. They are concerned with spirituality as a source of illumination and strength, how soul informs the mind and the will and encourages the social processes of reconciliation and community. This is an important emphasis because this is how soul becomes visible. In itself, soul is the invisible center of the person. It manifests

---

tion came over and over again like a pendulum 'What am I? What am I?' The words became a shout and then a whole scream of anger from a tense face and mouth. 'What am I? I am a bloody idiot who does not know what he is. Who cannot answer a simple question.' My cries got louder and louder. Rain and wind carried them back to me. This shuffling, shouting, scruffy figure in the stable punched at the air. Every muscle was tight. I was going to burst. . . . At the very moment of bursting frustration; at the very height of all the wind, rain, and fury, I was aware, quite softly, that I was actually keeping the answer at bay. Like an old and discreet friend, he had been patiently waiting to come in all this time. He came in and my whole body relaxed and jumped, felt good and warm. NOW I was now—the answer was NOW. I am/was/shall be everything which unfolds and moves, thinks, questions, and talks at that moment in time. It was far more than a purely intellectual realization—it bathed me with my goodness, everyone's goodness. Goodness happening now. I shouted happily, 'Now, now, now.' I and the question had become friends."

The following is spiritual reflection, a more intellectual expression, of the same dawning insight that soul is the essence of the human person. "Am I now able to answer the question which I was asking at the beginning of my inquiry? Can I say who am I? Nothing could be less sure. I have learned to recognize in the personality more or less profound levels. I have taken back properties to their own principles. But levels cover a center, and properties have an owner. I have pushed as far as possible my investigation without ever being able to get at something more than my belonging. To recognize them as mine, means to differentiate myself from them. I certainly am not either this body through which sensations come, and which I use for action, nor those tendencies, good or bad ones, that manifest through it. I can even see in the light of experience that I cannot be a body or an aggregate of bodies or a characteristic derived from some particular form of bodies. Those hypotheses which I am refusing were not false propositions, but meaningless affirmations. However, even if I cannot in any way get hold of myself, I nevertheless know that I am, and that I cannot doubt to be . . . If I wanted to speak more rigorously, I should than say I am I, expressing in this unusual way the fact that the I is always the subject. If I prefer to use a term which belongs both to common use and to the philosopher's language, I will not say, as is sometimes done, that I have a soul (which, to be precise, is contradictory, but that I am a soul." Gaston Berger, quoted in Roberto Assagioli, *The Act of Will* (New York: Penguin Books.)

itself by its effects in the more accessible dimensions of life, by its contributions to physical, mental, and social life. Since the presenting interests of health care in spirituality concern how the spiritual contributes to health, overall well-being, organizational excellence, and ethical living, this eye of the soul is of major concern.

In particular, this eye of the soul provides ultimate meaning and perspective. It is a big picture appraisal, seeing what is happening in its most comprehensive context. Alfred North Whitehead described entertaining ultimate perspectives as an airplane ride. You go high into the sky and see the land you just left from a heightened perspective. Then you return to the land with the benefit of the airplane view. Just what this benefit is, however, is often difficult to articulate. In Kenneth Pargament's study of religion and coping, he called this the transition from heaven to earth and suggested that coping is one way people could move from the "generalities of their faith" to the "dust of their trials."[39] Myles N. Sheehan, in reviewing a book on a Christian approach to ethics and medicine, pursues the same connection: "Likewise he (the author) left me, as a practitioner, continually wanting to know more about how Christian faith and the experience of the body (a theological, ultimate perspective) concretely express themselves in medical care and ethical concerns."[40] Once this eye of the soul is open, we see the world from a spiritual perspective. But this spiritual perspective is an ultimate point of view,

39. Kenneth I. Pargament, *The Psychology of Religion and Coping: Theory, Research, Practice* (New York: Guilford Press, 1997), pp. 163–66.
40. Myles N. Sheehan, "Who Decides?" *America* (October 2, 1999): 37-39.

and we must seek out the ways it influences our proximate dealings.

Others within health care stress the centrality of the Sacred or Spirit or God in any understanding of spirituality.[41] For them, talk of transcendence and meaning without an explicit awareness of the ground of transcendence and meaning reduces spirituality to immanent mental processes. In other words, they are focusing on the eye of the soul that peers into the eternal. They are concerned with our awareness of our communion with Ultimate Reality.

> What is important is that you become aware of something. Awareness is what we are after here. This awareness may have come suddenly and overwhelmingly, but it may also have come ever so gradually. My favorite image for this is the coming of spring. Sometimes spring comes suddenly, with a big bang. Yesterday it was still winter, but today spring is in the air. Spring came overnight. In other years, it comes so gradually that you can not even say when it came. A long drawn-out battle was going back and forth. But eventually it is spring. You do not know how it came, but all that matters is that spring is here. And so all that matters is that you eventually become aware deep within you of ultimate communion.[42]

---

41. See David B. Larson, James P. Sawyers, and Michael E. McCullough, *Scientific Research on Spirituality and Health* and Pargament, *Psychology of Religion and Coping.*

42. David Steindl-Rast, "Thoughts on Mysticism as Frontier of Consciousness Evolution" in *Human Survival and Consciousness Evolution,* ed. Stanislav Grof (Albany, New York: State University of New York Press, 1988), p. 97.

This emphasis is important. Whether a person becomes suddenly aware or gradually aware, the goal is to become aware. Inherited belief in God is meant to lead to an awareness of the relationship to God. This is the grounding for the spiritual life.

If the first eye of the soul provides an ultimate perspective on what is happening, this eye of the soul provides an ultimate identity. Spiritual teaching stresses that we have identities in all the dimensions, and at any given moment, there is a tendency to cling to one or the other. If we have a full head of hair, we tend to confer on it a "This is me" quality and designate ourselves as "He of the radiant locks." Or if we manage an "A" in economics, we quickly collapse ourselves into this academic glory and become "She of the great intellect." Or if we work as a chief operating officer in a marketing firm, one day we may find our attachment to this position so complete that we say to ourselves and others, as if nothing more could be said, "I am a COO." Of if we have had a powerful experience of being abandoned by someone we love, we may so internalize that single, transitory experience that we think of ourselves as "the rejected one." Or if we are successful at ingratiating ourselves with other people, we may come to know ourselves as "the charmer." At any given moment our identity slides, and we equate ourselves with a physical quality, a mental attribute, a social role, a significant experience, or a personality trait.

However, when we are aware of our communion with God, we have an ultimate identity. This identity relativizes the other identities and provides a place to stand, a place from which to act. Yet an ultimate identity raises the same questions as an ultimate perspective. How does this identity affect our other more proximate identities, identities rooted in personality, body, role, and behavior? How is the ultimate truth of who we are integrated into the proximate truths of who we are?

When people note this gap between the ultimate identity and perspective of the soul and the concrete dealings of life, they often do so to discredit soul consciousness. The criticism is predictable. Soul consciousness is otherworldly, not connected to body, mind, and society. It has no relevancy for people dedicated to the affairs and turmoils of the earth. Yet the gap between soul consciousness and the everyday living of health care operations is not a reason to dismiss spiritual considerations. Rather, it names the spiritual project. The spiritual project is to close the gap, to bring the spiritual into mind, body, and society. The spiritual does not seek to escape the world. It seeks to penetrate all aspects of the world.

In Christian faith, the Johannine Christ who is conscious he comes from God and is going to God and who knows that the Father (God as Love) has given all things into his hands washes the feet of his disciples. His consciousness of the spiritual brings him into the world of feet. In other words, in the language of theology the transcendent spiritual seeks to be immanent. Although our soul consciousness gives us an ultimate identity and perspective, it does not take us further away from the concrete world. It drives us toward it. When the two eyes of the soul are open, we are most committed and most creatively engaged in the things of earth.[43] In this sense,

---

43. See John Shea, "Challenges and Competencies: the Theological and Spiritual Aspects of Catholic Health Care Leadership," *Health Progress* (January-February, 2000).

the spiritual can be called a resource in the multiple struggles that surround the enterprises of human health and sickness. Of course, to understand this resource the nature of the spiritual must be explored.

Spirit as Resource

Lao Tzu, an ancient Chinese spiritual teacher, characterized Spirit in a series of provocative images.

> The Spirit of the Fountain dies not.
> It is called the Mysterious Feminine.
> The Doorway of the Mysterious Feminine is called the Root of Heaven-and-Earth.
> Lingering like gossamer, it has only a hint of existence.
> And yet when you draw upon it, it is inexhaustible.[44]

This imaginative and evocative spiritual text first explores the spiritual as an undying fountain, water that eternally springs up so human thirst can be slaked. The Johannine Jesus employs the same image. "The water I will give them will become a fountain of water within them, welling up into eternal life" (Jn. 4:14). Isaac of Nineveh develops the same image. "There is a love like a small lamp, which goes out when the oil is consumed; or like a stream, which dries up when it doesn't rain. But there is a love that is like a mighty spring gushing up out of the earth; it keeps flowing forever, and is inexhaustible."[45] Spirit is focused on human refreshment. This is not

---

44. Lao Tzu, *Tao Te Ching*. Book 1, VI.
45. Quoted in *The Enlightened Mind*, ed. Stephen Mitchell (New York: HarperCollins Publishers, 1991).

a fickle commitment or an intermittent desire. It is undying, an everlasting expression of the nature of the spiritual.

The text from Lao Tzu also images the spiritual as the mysterious feminine that gives life to all there is. The Book of Wisdom also uses the image of the feminine and characterizes her powers in a similar way: "Although she is but one, she can do all things, and while remaining in herself, she renews all things" (Wis. 7:27). The spiritual is its own reality ("remaining in herself"), yet it can go out to renew all things. The Book of Wisdom continues, "She passes into holy souls making them friends of God and prophets" (Wis. 7: 27). An essential characteristic of the spiritual is its ability to pass into "things" without displacing anything of that into which it has passed. Spirit can be completely present in nonspiritual realities without disturbing the integrity of those realities. Therefore, the spiritual not only gives life, it holds the spiritual and material worlds together. It is the root of heaven and earth, a connective reality, coupling what could easily be disjointed. In this sense, the spiritual is the ultimate flowing grace that creates the personal unity of the four dimensions. It weaves the physical, psychological, and social into one and grounds it in the transcendent source of all existence.

Therefore, the desire of Spirit is to be in a life-giving relationship with all things. Its nature is to give itself for the benefit of others. Paradoxically, according to the laws of the spiritual, this does not mean Spirit is diminished. It does not lose itself. Rather it grows in the act of self-giving. This is the strange, odd, uncanny way of the Spirit. It may be so unassuming that it only hints at existence, "yet when we draw on it, it is inexhaustible." This must be correctly understood. It is not that Spirit is an infinite reserve so no matter how much we take there is still something left. Rather it is in the very act of drawing on Spirit that it become inexhaustible. Its nature is to grow not only by giving but by being received by those to whom it gives itself. When we are receiving the flow of Spirit that is being given, there is an endlessness to it, an endlessness activated by our act of drawing.

Since Spirit desires to pass into us for our well-being, talking about it as a "resource" is appropriate. However, there is also a danger in this language. "Resource" can connote something at our disposal to be used as we wish. Humans have a reputation for being disrespectful toward resources, using them recklessly and in ways they were not intended. People have tried this with the spiritual. They have demanded Spirit heal a body or instantaneously change a social condition. They have tried to yoke the power of the spiritual to their egotistic ambitions and their most violent fantasies. Spirit does not allow itself to be used in these ways. It moves on, as the following story points out.

> The water of life, wishing to make itself known on the face of the earth, bubbled up in an artesian well and flowed without effort or limit. People came to drink of the magic water and were nourished by it, since it was so clean and pure and invigorating. But humankind was not content to leave things in this Edenic state. Gradually, they began to fence the well, charge admission, claim ownership of the property around it, make elaborate laws as to who could come to the well, put locks on the gates. Soon the well was the property of the powerful and the elite. The water was angry and offended; it stopped flowing and began to bubble up in another place. The people who owned the property around the first well were so

engrossed in their power systems and ownership that they did not notice that the water had vanished. They continued selling the nonexistent water; and few people noticed that the true power was gone. But some dissatisfied people searched with great courage and found the new artesian well. Soon that well was under the control of the property owners, and the same fate overtook it. The spring took itself to yet another place—and this has been going on throughout history.[46]

Spirit cannot be seized, possessed, or incorporated into the profit schemes of benighted people. It is always a resource on its own terms. The human spiritual project is to learn how to freely receive this resource and to freely give it.

The Caring Spiritual

Therefore, in the unfolding agenda of self-care, it is appropriate to think and plan about how to care for our bodies, minds, and intimate and social relationships. However, when it comes to the spiritual dimension, a different approach is needed. The spiritual is the deepest center of the person. It is the place from which we care; it is not an "object" we care for. We are essentially soul, the ability to receive Spirit and communicate it into all we are and all the world is. Therefore, it is more appropriate to say that the spiritual cares for us than to say we care for the spiritual.

Let me begin by saying that I think there is a big difference between "nourishing your soul" and "being nourished by your soul." We don't nourish our soul. Our soul nourishes us. We

_____

46. Quoted in Elkins, 23.

don't do something to our soul so much as have our soul do something to us. Our challenge as human beings is to open ourselves to receive this nourishment—to rekindle our connection with our spirit, the spirit that is always there waiting to nurture, heal, and direct our lives.[47]

In distinguishing between the locus and goal of spiritual disciplines, Philip Novak makes the same observation.

And when speaking of "spiritual disciplines" it is helpful to remember that the word "spiritual" points to the goal of the work and not to its actual locus. For it is not the spirit that needs discipline. "Spirit" or its equivalent in other traditions points to the unconditioned dimension of ourselves which dwells in a timeless union with the Real and which is to be discovered or uncovered by means of the disciplines.

The true locus of the spiritual, or as I prefer to call it, contemplative discipline, is the psyche, that interdependent network of conditioned structures which forms and informs our very states of consciousness, our identities and our varying notions of what counts as valuable and real. And contemplatives universally presuppose that the psyche is malleable. Consciousness and the structures which determine it thus comprise the pivot point between whomever we think we are and ultimate reality. Contemplative discipline aims at nothing less than the transformation of the undergirding structures of our consciousness so that their new formation allows

47. Jack Canfield, "Rekindling the Fires of Your Soul," in *Handbook For The Soul*, ed. Richard Carlso and Benjamin Shield, (Boston: Little Brown & Co., 1995) p. 87.

us to awaken from the sleep of bondage and to stay awake—
both for our own welfare and for that of the human community.[48]

Stephen Levine, in his work with spiritual healing, reinforces
the remarks of Canfield and Novak:

> I do not feel comfortable with the term spiritual healing be-
> cause it leads one to believe that the spirit can be injured.
> Which it cannot. It is the uninjured, the uninjurable, the
> boundarilessness of being, the deathless. So what is offered
> here is not a spiritual healing, but a healing into spirit.[49]

Once this "unconditioned dimension of ourselves which dwells
in a timeless union with the Real" is uncovered, its care floods
our being.

Therefore, traditional "care of the soul" involves working
with the mind and the structures of consciousness in order
to open into soul and Spirit. Once this happens, a reverse flow
occurs. Spirit gives itself into the soul, mind, body, and
world. When religious traditions talk of the grace or the loving kindness or the mercy of God, they are exploring this self-
giving quality of Spirit. And when they talk of the human
disposition of surrender or dependence or humility, they are
exploring the human capacity to open and receive from the

---

48. Philip Novak, "The Dynamic of Attention in Discipline," in *Ultimate
Reality and Spiritual Discipline*, ed. James Duerlinger (New York: Paragon
House Publishers, 1984) pp. 83–84.
49. Stephen Levine, *Healing Into Life and Death* (New York: Doubleday,
1987), p. 6.

Reality whose nature it is to give. This is the distinctiveness of the spiritual, and it has to be taken into account as we explore how it interacts with the physical, psychological, and social dimensions.

Conclusion

The spiritual interests emerging within health care will be pursued in terms of further and more sophisticated medical and organizational research, creative efforts at implementation, and sensitive managing of practical and theoretical resistance. As important as these factors are, they are not enough. There is also a need for a working knowledge of the spiritual that legitimates the spiritual interests and provides a direction for development. This working knowledge begins with an enhanced understanding of health care as attending to physical, psychological, social, and spiritual dimensions of the person who is living on a continuum of health and sickness. These dimensions are always present, interacting with one another and yet having their own distinctiveness. Intentional health care means we attend to all these dimensions of ourselves and others. However, because of the distinctiveness of the spiritual, we have to attend to it in a particular way. Attending to the spiritual entails going within to the soul space, opening both the eye that looks into Spirit and the eye that looks into the world, and learning how to receive and give Spirit. Spirit is a resource that grounds, guides, and transforms human projects. When patients, families, friends, medical caregivers, chaplains, leaders, employees, and ethical reflectors are interested in the spiritual, at a minimum they are interested in being aware and staying aware of this reality. How can we be in touch with this reality so we can let it do what is its nature to do—give Spirit to each fragile and vulnerable human person? Spiritualities are how we stay in touch, how we open to what is there.

PART THREE

WELCOMING AND DEVELOPING SPIRITUALITIES

□ □ ■ □

Although it is 6:00 a.m. and still dark, the parking lot of the hospital is already filling up. In an hour only the far lots will be available. People are filing from their cars and meeting up with others who are getting off buses. They are all moving toward the hospital, its many windows spilling light into the last darkness before the day.

Who are these people?

Some are patients on a fourteen-hour fast, hoping to be first in line for blood testing. Some are patients coming for day surgery, believing they will sleep in their own beds tonight. Some are family and friends of patients—a wife who left the hospital late last night is now returning, a son who, every morning before he goes to work, visits his father in intensive care, a clergy person who was notified an hour ago that one of the parishioners had been admitted last night. Others are medical and nonmedical caregivers—nurses on day shift, doctors who need to fill in charts and visit patients before the rush begins, social workers who couldn't sleep and decided to come in early.

Later in the day they will be joined by others. More social workers, volunteers, and the administrative staff will begin arriving about eight. The CEO has a 8:30 meeting with those who report directly to her. Throughout the day there will be a flow of patients in and out of the hospital and adjacent medical center. Although all the people entering and exiting the buildings are involved in the enterprise of receiving and delivering health care services, they are there for different reasons and are in different mental and emotional states. Throughout the day, these diverse interests and states will be continuously interacting.

Upon entering this intricately structured social environment, these people are immediately assigned roles—patient, visitor, nurse, intake coordinator, doctor, engineer, lab technician, human resource manager, and so on. These roles set boundaries, determining what people expect and how they will relate to one another. Some of the rules of these roles are written down. There are statements of patients' rights, doctors' responsibilities, and job descriptions for everyone from volunteer to CEO. There are also unwritten rules—assumptions about how things are done, tacit agreements about what is appropriate and what is inappropriate, personal limits resulting from previous experiences in a health care environment. These unwritten rules are often the hidden determinants of inner attitudes and outer behavior. No one enters a health care setting without simultaneously taking on a role and playing by some rules.

Today these roles and rules are changing. For example, the patient-doctor relationship is considerably different than it was in the immediate past. The patient has more say in how his or her disease will be treated, and in some cases, insurance plans have more say than either the doctor or the patient. The roles are still there, but the rules and how they are being played out are changing. Health care settings are thick with rules, roles, responsibilities, and system considerations that are in flux, and many think that in the current volatile atmosphere of contemporary health care, change is the only certainty.

Spiritual People

Those people trudging into the hospital also bring with them varying capacities for spiritual awareness, a wide range of abilities to open to the spiritual and to see things from a spiritual point of view. During the course of the day, these capacities will be tapped. They will come into play in the midst of the rules, roles, responsibilities, and systems. The deeply personal will emerge to influence the socially structured relationships. This reflects a core spiritual teaching: people are more than their roles. Their participation in the spiritual dimension makes them transcendent to any roles they may play in various social dramas. This spiritual capacity of being more will eventually and in unforeseeable ways enter into the organized and reorganized delivery of health care.

Of course, the spiritual capacities of people vary greatly. When the spiritual is seen as a dimension of the human, it automatically becomes a human potential. It is not just a "given," but a "given" that can be developed. Just as the physical, psychological, and social are developed differently by different people, so spiritual development is a continuum with some people at the low end and some people at the high end.[1] For example, when Sister Thea Bowman was told she had cancer, she responded, "So now it's my turn." Her life-long spiritual practice had awakened in her a profound sense of solidarity with the human condition. She could see and evaluate suffering and death from the soul space. Contrast this with the often heard response when confronted with the news of cancer, "Why me?" The first response reflects the spiritual awareness of communion; the second response reflects the fantasy of separation and exemption. Sister Thea was able to access her spiritual resources.

Of course, one expects that professional religious, chaplains, and clergy will have developed their capacity to enter the soul space, be open to the spiritual, and reflect the spiritual in what they say and do. Yet, on the whole, social roles are not indicators of spiritual development. The people most in touch with the spiritual dimension and thereby most able to communicate it may not be at the top of the social and organizational ladder. Dawna Markova, for instance, tells a

1. The fact of spiritual development always raises the question of elitism. Will the more highly developed use this fact as a social advantage to the detriment of others? These are many responses to this "envisioned situation." One of the more interesting is that spiritual development entails relativizing the ego and its insatiable demands for protection and promotion. Those who are highly developed spiritually do not seek power over others. Instead, they offer whatever they have to contribute to the well-being of others. The goal of spiritual development is not social position but spiritual service.

story about a lady who cleaned the floor of the hospital where she was a patient.

One night she reached out and put her hand on the top of my shoulder. I'm not usually comfortable with casual touch, but her hand felt so natural being there. It happened to be one of the few place in my body that didn't hurt. I could have sworn she was saying two words with every breath, one of the inhale, one of the exhale: "As . . . Is . . . As . . . Is . . . "

On her next visit, she looked at me. No evaluation, no trying to figure me out. She just looked and saw me. Then she said simply, "You're more than the sickness in that body." . . . I kept mumbling those words to myself throughout the following day. "I'm more than the sickness in this body. I'm more than the suffering in this body." I remember the voice clearly. It was rich, deep, full, like maple syrup in the spring. . . .

I reached out for her hand. It was cool and dry. I knew she wouldn't let go. She continued, "You're not the fear in that body. You're more than that fear. Float on it. Float above it. You're more than that pain." I began to breathe a little deeper, as I did when I wanted to float in a lake. I remembered floating in Lake George when I was five, floating in the Atlantic Ocean at Coney Island when I was seven, floating in the Indian Ocean off the cost of Africa when I was twenty-eight. Without any instruction from me, this Jamaican guide had led me to a source of comfort that was wider and deeper than pain and fear.[2]

---

2. Dawna Markova, *No Enemies Within*, quoted in Frederic and Mary Ann Brussat, *Spiritual Literacy* (New York: Simon & Schuster, 1996), pp. 396–97.

This spiritually developed cleaning lady became an ad hoc spiritual companion to a patient. She instructed her in spiritual practices that brought the woman's consciousness into the soul space where she realized her transcendent spiritual identity—"You're more than the pain in that body." This realization brought great comfort and peace.

From Spiritual Communities

The cleaning lady did not learn that spiritual practice by mopping floors. (Although for someone this spiritually developed, mopping floors is probably spiritual activity.) She had a history of spiritual development, a soul story, that she brought to work that day. So it is with most of the people who enter health care settings day after day. If they have developed spiritual capacities, most probably they have developed and nurtured them outside the health care setting. They may be practicing Muslims, Christians, Jews, Hindus, Buddhists, or so forth, and these religious affiliations may have made them familiar with the reality of soul. Or they may have developed this capacity from participation in psychotherapy, the human potential movement, or any number of other activities and communities. However it has occurred, spiritual awareness is a potential that people have learned to actualize along the way. When they enter health care settings, they bring that ability with them.

From his study of spirituality within organizations, Frederic Craigie concluded "that developing spirituality and spiritual wellness in organizations is primarily a matter of cultivating that which is already there, rather than introducing or teaching something that is absent."[3] However, "that which is already there" came from someplace. Although organized health care settings are appropriate places for spiritual activity, they are not the home of spiritual activity. The principal places of spiritual nurture are elsewhere. Although each person has his or her own individual spirituality, they usually belong to a spiritual community that supports and legitimates their spiritual interest and sensitivity. These communities and traditions are essential for spiritual development. They provide encouragement for the spiritual search, wisdom about the "ups and downs" of the spiritual path, established leadership and spiritual guidance, and commonly shared experiences of spiritual nurture and renewal. If health care is interested in the spiritual development of both patients and associates, it must help people stay in contact with these communities.

Carrying Spiritualities: Beliefs, Stories, and Practices

Spiritual people from spiritual communities carry with them spiritualities. Spiritualities are composed of beliefs, stories, and practices that focus on the spiritual dimension and its subtle interactions with the physical, psychological, and social dimensions. These beliefs, stories, and practices are not ends in themselves. They are in the service of spiritual consciousness. They are meant to bring awareness into the soul

---

3. Frederic C. Craigie, Jr., "The Spirit and Work: Observations About Spirituality and Organizational Life," *Journal of Psychology and Christianity* 18 (1999): 43–53.

space, the deepest center of consciousness, and to facilitate seeing and acting from that space. Spiritualities are the creations of spiritual people for the express purpose of staying in touch with the spiritual, both in themselves and in their situations.

This point about the goal of spiritualities is important. Spiritualities do not directly contribute to the repairing or healing of particular situations. However, since spiritualities are often brought forward in pressing circumstances (for example, people often suggest prayer as a last-ditch response after everything else has been tried), an expectation arises that the beliefs, stories, and practices will have an immediate impact on the situation. This expectation is misplaced. Spiritualities directly contribute to the repair and healing of our relationship to the spiritual by helping us consciously attend to it.[4] Once we are in conscious contact with the spiritual, it may become a resource to creatively address whatever is happening in the situation. However, this alleviation of the situation is always mediated by the people who engage the spiritualities and so center themselves in the spiritual and open themselves to its direction. Spiritualities are first _for_ people and then _through_ people for the betterment of situations.

Spiritualities are irreducibly individual. A person may belong to and participate in a Catholic, Hindu, or Islamic religious community, yet this alone cannot predict her or his

---

4. For a clear presentation of this insight, see "Beyond Ego: An Interview with Hameed Ali," *Common Boundary* (November/December 1999), pp. 18–24.

spirituality.[5] They have probably selected one or two beliefs from these traditions, have a particular sacred story that they prize and consult, and engage in one or another religious practice, although these particular beliefs, stories, and practices may not be the ones the officials of the tradition consider central. Also, they have gathered beliefs, stories, and practices from their individual experiences and blended these with what they have learned from their religious traditions. These collective traditions and personal experience are the two sources that people draw on for the beliefs, stories, and practices that comprise their spiritualities. The result is a unique combination of influences that structure their consciousness in a certain way. Therefore, the only way to discover a person's spirituality and the effect it is having on their consciousness is to listen carefully as they reveal it.

For example, a patient may believe God is present no matter how bad things get. He connects this with a song he always sang in church, "My God is a rock in a weary land, in a weary land, in a weary land. My God is a rock in a weary land, shelter in a time of storm." He remembers his grandmother told him stories about the Depression when they had nothing but faith to keep them going and every morning they prayed for strength. He has taken up that practice. He prays every morning, "Lord, give me the strength to get through the day." The question is, how does this spirituality, this combination of belief, story, and practice, shape his con-

---

5. See David McCurdy, "Religion and Spirituality in the Clinical Setting: Ethical Challenges and Opportunities," *Insights: Ethics Newsletter* (Winter 1999).

sciousness and open him to the spiritual dimension of human interactions?

Or a nurse may believe that because everybody is related to God and because God is behind it all, everybody is related to everybody else. She had a dream once that reinforced this belief. She dreamt that her sister, who lived two thousand miles away, was sick. In the morning she called and found out her sister had pneumonia and was in the hospital. What she dreamed was actual. She was connected to her sister in a way that was not completely conscious. She concluded, in what she herself admits was a wild leap, that there is an invisible network of communication throughout the universe. She used that network to pray for her sister. Now she prays for all her patients. She does not pray for specific things, like better health or that more people would come and visit. She prays for them in a simple and direct way, asking God to open them to healing. She thinks that is a better way. The question is, how does this spirituality, this combination of belief, story, and practice shape her consciousness and open her to the spiritual dimension of human interactions?

Or an upper-management executive may believe that, down deep, people want to help other people. This is basic. She remembers how she found this out about herself. Her boss turned to her and said half-jokingly and half-seriously, "Face it, Joan, you're a do-gooder." Once she faced it, she was happier. She often begins department meetings with, "Let's see what we can do to make things better for people." Colleagues are not sure whether to take her seriously. She often supports the staff by reminding them how what they do affects other people, even though they do not immediately see it. Although she says she is not very religious, she considers this her spiritual practice—reminding herself and others that down deep they are driven by a desire to help. The question is, how does this spirituality, this combination of belief, story, and practice, shape her consciousness and open her to the spiritual dimension of human interactions? Spiritualities are the stethoscopes people possess to hear the pulse of the spiritual in each experience and in every situation. The more people explore spiritual beliefs, tell and re-tell spiritual stories, and engage in spiritual practices, the more developed their spiritual consciousness becomes. In the language of spiritual traditions, they develop eyes to see and ears to hear. What they see and hear is the spiritual, not as a "thing apart," but as deep activity arising and transforming the social interactions of health care.

A Welcoming Organization

Spiritual people from spiritual communities carrying spiritualities arrive within an organized medical system of health care delivery. Will the medical center be hospitable to this dimension of the people it serves? If the organization is going to welcome spiritualities, it will have to marshall appropriate and convincing reasons for doing so and also work out the practicalities.

A health care organization may welcome spiritualities for many reasons:

- because the majority of patients and employees want it and it may increase employee morale, patient satisfaction, and market share;

- because the organization is committed to holistic care and the spiritual is included in that comprehensive approach;
- because the organization is faith-based, and welcoming the spiritual is a logical extension of its identity and mission;
- because medical and organizational research suggests that the inclusion of the spiritual contributes to the excellence of medical care and organizational well-being.

Big-picture reasons for welcoming the spiritual are needed as a context for the difficult and long-haul organizational effort this welcoming will entail.

The "why" of welcoming always unfolds into more intricate and sensitive practicalities. How will the welcoming go on?

- Will spiritual screening tools be added to intake forms? If they are added, what questions will be asked and what will be done with them?
- Will physicians and nurses inquire about a patient's spirituality and be prepared to respond to what they find?
- Will the organization reconsider its policies around productivity and performance to include spiritual concerns?
- Will staff pray with patients if they are invited to do so?
- How will the spiritualities of different faiths be handled, especially if the health care organization is of one particular faith?
- How will proselytizing and religious bickering be avoided?

- Education in spirituality and health will be needed, but how will it go on and how will it be evaluated?
- How will leadership encourage the spirituality of employees and associates so that they will be able to welcome the spiritualities of patients?
- Does this inclusion of the spiritual involve new responsibilities for chaplains and pastoral care personnel?
- Are all spiritualities welcome? What if a spirituality clashes with the health care organization's values of what is considered the most beneficial medical treatment?

The ultimate test of welcoming spiritualities will come down to how the welcoming is done and who is doing it. In many situations, it is assumed that those who think welcoming spiritualities is a good idea will not be those who actually do it. Therefore, the usual organizational division between those who decide and those who implement will cause the usual problem—the spirit of welcoming will be lost and in its place will be wooden compliance with a new rule sent down from above. The decision to go public and welcome spiritualities leads inevitably to questions about how to change organizational culture and behavior.

Background Spiritualities and Foreground Spiritualities

There is more to say about welcoming spiritualities into health care than noting the difficulties and possibilities of efforts at inclusion. The spiritualities that people bring into health care settings have been developed in other settings, most notably within religious traditions and communities. This means they have been created and amended in communal settings. The beliefs are often convictions that have been hammered out in the long history of the community. These beliefs usually focus on the spiritual itself, not the spiritual as it relates to health care. They may be beliefs about the nature of the Divine, the dynamics of sin and redemption, what happens at death, the possibility of after life salvation, and the end-of-the-world. The spiritual stories are also community oriented. They may be about the founder—Abraham and Sarah, Moses, Jesus, Mohammed, Gotama—or about key holy people within the history of the tradition. Also, the practices are those of the people gathered together, geared toward a community of believers rather than individuals outside the community in specific settings. These communal practices are rituals that incorporate beliefs and stories and provide the ongoing spiritual nurture for the people.

These community rituals are scheduled for certain times and certain places. These times and places become sacred times and sacred places because the community, in an explicit way, focuses on the spiritual dimension of life and, in most traditions, on its relationship to the Divine Source. For example, there is Sabbath observance in synagogue or temple for Jews or Sunday worship in church for Christians. However, this official community gathering is only one day a week and, then, only for an hour or two. The question that naturally arises is how to allow the deeper consciousness of Sabbath and Sunday time to influence the consciousness of the rest of the week. "The resacralization of the world must finally make a difference in our everyday lives, not just in some split-off part that we define as our spiritual time or space. All space is potentially sacred space, all time is potentially sacred time."[6] This struggle to extend spiritual consciousness to times and places that are not officially designated as sacred has been called "living the faith" or the "sanctification of everyday life" or "putting faith into practice."

One way of sanctifying everyday life is to create spiritualities around the major stages and landmark transition moments of life—birth, adolescence, leave-taking, marriage, menopause, midlife, aging, and death. This task continues with even greater particularity by shaping spiritualities around the repeatable and essential elements of ordinary life—waking up, eating, working, being with others, words, movements, simple pleasures, going to sleep.[7] These two sets of spiritualities make spiritual consciousness a possible companion to every human experience. As important as the communally shared background spiritualities are, it is often difficult to connect them with the nitty-gritty interactions of daily work and relationships. If the spiritual dimension is to enter consciousness in the ordinary experiences of life, there is a need for foreground spiritualities, for spiritualities geared to what is happening.

This is especially true in health care. Whatever foreground spiritualities people already have and whatever foreground spiritualities will be developed, they must contribute in two

---

6. Michael Lerner, *Jewish Renewal: A Path to Healing and Transformation* (New York: Grosset/Putnam, 1994), p. xxxvii.
7. These categories are taken from Philip Zaleski and Paul Kaufman, *Gifts of the Spirit: Living The Wisdom of the Great Religious Traditions* (San Francisco: HarperSanFrancisco, 1997).

ways. First, they must awaken spiritual consciousness in the midst of the social interactions of health care. In other words, they must help the person move interiorly into the soul space. This move is not a way of leaving the outer world. It is a way of finding a luminous space in order to be present to the outer world in a more complete way. Second, foreground spiritualities must help the person flow out from this space. They must help spirit inform behavior. The ultimate goal of foreground spiritualities is to bring the resources of the soul space into the outer world and change that world along lines suggested by the spiritual. To put this another way, the sanctification of the everyday is the place where spiritualities and moral living come together.

Foreground Spiritualities and Values

In this way, foreground spiritualities connect with and support individual and organizational values. Values play an important role in most health care organizations. They occupy a middle ground between convictions and concrete actions. Values—for example, respect, excellence, compassion, and collaboration—are grounded in some convictions. These convictions can be about such things as the nature of the human person, the dynamics of healing, the workings of society, and the role of medicine. However, these convictions are assumed more than they are stated. They are seldom explicitly brought forth, which allows people to "buy into" the values on whatever convictional grounds are comfortable for them. For example, a Christian health care organization may have "respect" as one of its guiding values. The official organizational grounding for it may be the conviction that the human person is made in the image of God. However, a given employee may espouse the value of respect because without it "society would fall apart" or because he or she follows the golden rule of doing unto others as you would have them do unto you. The middle position of values allows people to embrace them with whatever grounding is convincing to them.

This middle position of values also drives one of health care's most urgent projects: what do these values mean and how do you implement them? It is one thing to state the values and quite another to live them. In fact, because the discrepancy between saying and doing is often so great, many people become cynical. They see values talk as a cover for policies and behaviors that are heedless of the very values that supposedly guide the organization. If values are not operationalized, they become a sham. Therefore, the drive to implement the values is crucial to the identity and integrity of any given health care organization.

One help in the effort to implement values is to spell out behaviors that embody them. For example, consider an organization that characterizes itself as showing respect for all people no matter what their condition or circumstances. Part of the organization is a retirement living community. Concerned people have drawn up some tips on showing respect for the elderly.

1. Use Mr., Mrs., or Miss with last names unless residents invite you to call them by their first name.
2. Try to be the same height as the older person (e.g., if they are in a wheelchair, pull up a chair; if they are in bed, sit down beside them).
3. Address questions directly to them, not indirectly through caregivers.

The list goes on. Yet, as helpful as these tips are, they are not enough.

It is always a person who acts. Therefore, where they are "at" internally when they engage in these behaviors is important. Even the most objectively respectful action can be undercut by an inner, unmindful or disrespectful attitude. All the tips begin with words such as use, try, start speak, touch, accept; the person is initiating an action. With what consciousness is the action being performed? This is the concern of foreground spiritualities. Their ambition is to evoke an appropriate awareness in the inner world so the actions in the outer world will truly communicate respect. Spiritualities target the whole person who acts.

Also, there are not enough "tips for respect" to cover all the things that could possibly happen. There are always unforeseen situations. In fact, the actual unruly flow of life has more unpredictability than predictability. These unforeseen situations cannot be envisioned and plotted out beforehand. There must be an internalized sense of respect that will surface and find a creative expression in the unforeseen situation. Frederic Craigie tells the story of an oncology nurse who was working with a cancer patient. The patient was experiencing many painful losses and was on the verge of despair. The nurse was not able to get the man to talk at any length. Not knowing what to do, she invited him to go for a walk in the garden outside the facility. On the ground was a dead butterfly. Without comment she picked up the butterfly and gave it to him. This opened the man up and he began to talk about his life. Craigie comments,

Taking a walk and picking up the butterfly are creative processes that are not deduced from a model. Certainly there is no psychotherapy algorithm which says, "go outside, find a dead animal, and give it to the patient." To the extent that what we as would-be healers do is inductive and creative, it places a premium on our ability to be open to inspiration, or in-spiriting. It places a premium on our spiritual well-being, and on our ability to be receptive to the movement of the Spirit in using us in sometimes unforeseen ways as agents of change and healing.[8]

In the last analysis, implementing values is most effectively and consistently done by people who have internalized those values and integrated them into the way they see and act.

Many of the individual and organizational values within health care are words that have spiritual resonance—respect, compassion, empathy, cooperation, responsibility, partnership, equality, excellence. These are intrinsic qualities of people when they are in touch with the deeper level of the spiritual within themselves and in the situation. The ambition of foreground spiritualities is to keep people conscious of spirit as they deal with flesh. The premise is simple: people in touch with the spiritual are more excellent in every way. They embody the values that are essential to medicine and healing in an easy and creative way, a way appropriate to the gracefulness of the spiritual.

I think people in health care settings have intuitively developed foreground spiritualities. Although these spiritualities have beliefs and stories attached to them, the focus is on

---

8. Craigie, "Spirit and Work," 50.

practices. Practices are a combination of inner and outer actions that bring consciousness into the soul space and out of the soul space into the world. A patient in a waiting room interiorly prays the Lord's Prayer. A doctor washes her hands and recites a Jewish prayer of purification. A nurse pauses before she begins her shift and says, "Each one is brother and sister to me." The executive team uses silence throughout their meeting in order to remember the forest as they plunge into the trees. A chaplain sits with a dead body before it is taken away. He does not know why he does this; but he does this. As he sits there, he does not think. He just sits there. All he knows is that it is a practice of humility before mystery, a mystery easily forgotten. The mystery is not easily forgotten because it is not present, it is easily forgotten because it is so present it becomes routine. The danger is that we steel ourselves against death. So he sits in silence, the noise of the hospital floor surrounding him. It is his practice. For all he knows, people are off in some other spot engaging in their practice. The suspicion is that people in health care settings develop multiple, individual practices to open themselves to the spiritual. They do this to stay spiritually healthy in an environment that paradoxically has ongoing invitations into spiritual depth and also ongoing invitations into soul blindness.

There are three foreground spiritualities that might be especially helpful for the people and situations of health care—a spirituality of self-remembering, a spirituality of knowledge, and a spirituality of compassion. These spiritualities are not meant to replace the background spiritualities with their strong sense of tradition and community. Rather, they are meant to enhance and extend the contact with the spiritual in the tradition of "living the faith" or "sanctifying daily life." But if they are to do this, they must be related to the dynamics of the particular "daily life" they are trying to sanctify. Therefore, these three foreground spiritualities tap into and explore some of the pervasive features of health care settings.

A Spirituality of Self-Remembering

Health care settings are places of constant activity and, at times, great pressure. Both direct service and support areas have emergency procedures in place. People can be drawn into one high stress situation after another. They also can be in contact with other people who are anxious, angry, or loud. Everyone has expectations, responsibilities, and time lines. Lunch is a luxury. In this rushed and demanding atmosphere, there is also a tendency on the part of patients and staff to reduce people to their sickness. "There's a gallbladder in 205." Even when we know it is Mrs. Smith with the gallbladder, we forget and think in terms of what she is "in" for—gallbladder. With so much to do, many people must act in close coordination to accomplish things. Hence, clear role definitions and minutely spelled out responsibilities are a must. Yet with these comes the option to lose oneself, to lose sight of the person who is acting. In these dynamics of health care, a spirituality of self-remembering may be appropriate.

A story that helps to focus the project of self-remembering is, "What is the world like?"

God and a man are walking down the road. The man asks God, "What is the world like?"

God replies, "I cannot talk when I am thirsty. If you could get me a drink of cool water, we could discuss what the world is like. There is a village nearby. Go and get me a drink."

The man goes into the village and knocks at the door of the first house. A comely young woman opens the door. His jaw drops, but he manages to say, "I need a glass of cool water."

"Of course," she says, smiling, "but it is midday. Would you care to stay for some food?"

"I *am* hungry." he says, looking over his shoulder. "And your offer of food is a great kindness."

He goes in and the door closes behind him.

Thirty years goes by. The man who wanted to know what the world was like and the woman who offered him food have married and raised five children. He is a respected merchant and she is an honored woman of the community. One day a terrible storm comes in off the ocean and threatens their life. The merchant cries out, "Help me, God."

A voice from the midst of the storm says, "Where is my cup of cold water?"

This story reflects a universal spiritual teaching. We have a tendency to lose ourselves in worldly pursuits. The world is a series of invitations, responsibilities, tasks, and duties. Although we are obliged to engage them, they monopolize our time and consciousness. As we are dealing with them, we forget who we are. The deeper dimensions of ourselves are neglected. The essential mission of acknowledging and serving God has been ignored.

When we become aware we have neglected this important aspect of who we are, we fantasize we must leave the world in order to attend to God, to bring the long-awaited cup of cool water. A false dichotomy is set up—either God or the world. However, the calling of most people is not to choose between God and the world but to bring the two together, to integrate the spiritual and the social. In the time-honored spiritual proverb, we are meant to be "in the world, but not of it." We have to go about what we have to do without losing sight of who we are. This is the spiritual project of self-remembering.

The spiritual teaching of self-remembrance focuses on the inner space of outer actions. This is not the same as seeking out and exploring motivation. It is not about why we are doing something, but where we are at as we do it. There seems to be an infinite number of inner spaces that become the atmosphere of our words and deeds. For example, often we are simply missing. We are not there as we act. We are remembering something that has happened in the past or are thinking about something that is about to happen in the future. Or we "steel ourselves" and act. We are doing something unpleasant and so we "harden our hearts" and do it. Or we do something because we have said we would do it, only now we wish we had not committed ourselves. We are a hostage to a past promise. And as a hostage we act. Or we do something because we have always done it. We are habituated, and we proceed mindlessly through the day. From this perspective, many actions are mindless, done without attention.[9]

---

9. Of course, mindfulness is a spiritual practice that has been applied to every aspect of human life. For example, see Mylas and Jon Kabat-Zinn, *Everyday Blessings: The Inner Work of Mindful Parenting* (New York: Hyperion, 1997).

Spiritual teachers suggest we clear away all this inner debris and center ourselves, deepening consciousness into the soul space. Once it is there and the two eyes of the soul are open, we should go about our work. This inner centering is what makes an action spiritual. In a conventional framework, spiritual actions are words and deeds explicitly directed toward God, for example, prayers, confessions of faith, and religious rituals. In this framework, a spiritual action is one that comes from a spiritual space. The action itself may be diapering a baby, taking a blood pressure, listening to a fellow patient, holding a hand, or inquiring about a condition. But doing it from the soul space imbues the action with certain qualities.

One quality of spiritual actions is that they uncover the soul space in others. Actions from the soul space invite others into their own soul space. In other words, there is a meeting at a deeper level.

I have a friend, a chemotherapy nurse in a children's cancer ward, whose job is to pry for any available vein in an often emaciated arm to give infusions of chemicals that sometimes last as long as twelve hours and which are often quite discomforting to the child. He is probably the greatest pain-giver the children meet in their stay in the hospital. Because he has worked so much with his own pain, his heart is very open. He works with his responsibilities in the hospital as a "laying on of hands with love and acceptance." There is little in him that causes him to withdraw, that reinforces the painfulness of the experience for the children. He is a warm, open space which encourages them to trust whatever they feel. And it is he whom the children most often ask for at the time they are dying. Although he is the main pain-giver, he is also the main love-giver.[10]

This is a powerful testimony. His inner work with his own pain allows him a way of "working with his responsibilities." He draws blood from the soul space, an inner space of love and acceptance. Therefore, he invites the children into that space, a space that does not reinforce the painfulness and suffering.

Another quality of the soul space is that it invents ways to better situations. I was told a story about an explosive situation in a drug and rehabilitation center that points out the creativity of the soul space. A strong, tall man with a baseball bat entered the reception area. He was drunk and began shouting obscenities and banging the bat on the desks of the secretaries and admitting personnel. They jumped back and tried to get as far away from him as possible. One ran into the back room and phoned the police. As the woman who told me this story put it, "Suddenly the older woman who was the director of the center appeared." She walked right up to the screaming man who was waving the bat. She ducked under his arms and wrapped her arms around his chest. In a heartfelt voice she repeated over and over again, "Oh, you poor man! Oh, you poor man!" They stood together in that strange embrace for a while. Then the man began to sob. The woman led him to a chair. He slumped into it. In a few minutes the police came and took him away.

10. Ram Dass and Paul Gorman, *How Can I Help?* (New York: Knopf, 1985). pp. 86–87.

Perhaps this story is overly dramatic, but it shows the creativity, courage, and comfort of actions that flow from the spiritual center. Actions from this source almost always exhibit engagement instead of fear and avoidance. The outside world does not dictate the terms on which the person will act. The predictable response to violence is flight or countervioleence. In the story, the woman responds with disarming compassion. Her inner freedom was greater than the outer coercion to violence. Spiritual actions not only come from the soul space, they carry the love of that space into complex, highly charged situations.

Therefore, self-remembering is the ability not to lose touch with soul as you become more in touch with the world. Some spiritual traditions name this ability "contemplation in action." Adepts strive to master these "twin touches," this dual consciousness. They remain centered in the inner world as they act in the outer world. Obviously, this is an ideal. For most of us, self-remembering is an ongoing process tightly linked with self-forgetting. We lose it and regain it and lose it again. Self-remembering is not something we accomplish. It is a path we are on.

Three practices are helpful along the spiritual path of self-remembering. The first is redoing. When we lose "it" (our sense of ourself and what we are really about) and then later regain "it," it is important to go back to the people and situations where we lost it and redo what happened. "Losing it" takes many forms. Sometimes it is being inattentive, perfunctory, even dismissive. At other times, it is internalizing the negative tones of the outer situation and joining in its destructive path. When this happens, we can return and redo. Spiritual development means learning the path of repentance and finding the voice of conversion. But it must be a simple voice, modest in religious rhetoric. It must witness to the fact that the negative past can be reclaimed and reconstructed in a better way.

The second practice is pausing. We live in a fast-paced society and in many situations, especially in health care settings, it is justified, even necessary, to act in haste. However, a steady diet of speed usually means the mind races and we lose the inner concentration of the soul space. At times like these, it is necessary to pause. The pause allows us to go inside, recenter, observe the mind, and, most importantly, choose our words and actions. Pausing is a practice that moves us from reaction to response. The outer situation has not mindlessly triggered our words and deeds. We have moved to the resources of the soul. Within that space and out of that space we formulate a response infused by Spirit. In fast-paced situations pausing is the prerequisite of intentional living.

A third practice is inner listening. This practice takes pausing a step further. It is not only pulling out of the outer world to recenter and choose a response. It is centering and dwelling in such a way that the deeper levels can emerge into consciousness with both their wisdom and folly. Inner listening usually takes a longer time than pausing. However, when insights and actions that were not previously seen and that seem particularly appropriate to the situation at hand arise from the soul space, we have one of the surest experiences of the spiritual as an inner resource. People who make inner listening a consistent part of their life will often confidently remark, "The words and actions will be given." To those of us accustomed to only rational analysis, intervention, and evaluation, this level of trust seems unwarranted. The people a little further down this particular spiritual path smile and say, "Try it."

A Spirituality of Knowledge
The following story from the Buddhist tradition lays out a problem of the mind. Although this problem is shared by everyone, it becomes particularly evident in health care settings. A spirituality of knowledge alertness begins by noticing this problematic feature of how the mind functions.

A young widower, who loved his five-year-old son very much, was away on business. Bandits came, burned down his whole village, and took away his son. When the man returned, he saw the ruins and panicked. He took the charred corpse of an infant to be his own child, and he began to pull his hair and beat his chest, crying uncontrollably. He organized a cremation ceremony, collected the ashes, and put them in a very beautiful velvet bag. Working, sleeping, eating—he always carried the bag of ashes with him.

One day his real son escaped from the robbers and found his way home. He arrived at his father's new cottage at midnight, and knocked at the door. Inside the young father was still carrying the bag of ashes, and crying.

He asked, "Who is there?"
And the child answered, "It's me, Papa. Open the door. It's your son."
In his agitated state of mind the father thought that some mischievous boy was making fun of him. He shouted at the child to go away, and he continued to cry.

The boy knocked again and again, but the father refused to let him in. Some time passed, and finally the child left.

The Buddha comments on this story, "Sometime, somewhere you take something to be the truth. If you cling to it so much, when the truth comes in person and knocks at your door, you will not open it."[11]

This story points to the dark side of holding knowledge to be true. We may become attached to what we think we know in such a way that it keeps us from knowing more. It is not so much the knowledge as our attachment to it that closes us down rather than opens us up to the actual. This predicament is captured in the Buddhist phrase, "In the mind of the expert there is only one possibility: in the mind of the beginner there are many." We are urged to cultivate beginner's mind. This is not a call to abandon the pursuit of knowledge but an invitation to set up a relationship with the mind and what it knows, to open a space between who we are and what we know.

Setting up a relationship with the mind is the natural consequence of pulling consciousness into the soul space. When the eye of the soul that looks into the world has been opened, the first "thing" that comes into view are the workings of the mind. We are usually surprised by what we see. The immediate discovery is that the mind has a life of its own. Things happen and the mind moves. Things don't happen and the mind moves. Although we may cultivate the illusion that we are controlling our thoughts, most likely our thoughts think

---

11. Told in Thich Nhat Hanh, *Being Peace* (Parallax Press, 1996).

themselves.[12] Our minds are active independent of our attention to them. In fact, when we try to pay attention to something, we find we are distracted by the noise of the mind. The mind has its own agenda, and it is avidly pursuing it. We "bump" into our minds as obstacles to our deeper desires to attend to something else. This chronic "chatter and cinema" of the mind is often imaged as tapes. The mind is a tape library and when the tapes start playing, they steal consciousness away. When we set up a relationship to the mind, we immediately face the question of how to make its obvious energy serve our deeper purposes.

This spiritual project begins with exercising disindentification.[13] We try not to identify with the contents of the mind, and so we are not taken down paths we have not chosen. In a frustrated voice we may say, "I can't get it out of my mind." On one level, we know it is "my" mind, and so it should be under "my" control. But on another level, we recognize that we are bound to the information or perspective the mind is presenting or the tape it is playing. The fact is that the mind has us more than we have it. It is said that the mind makes a good servant but a bad master. When we are so tightly tied to its automatic firings that we cannot free ourselves, the truth can knock on the door and we will send it away because of our identification with what we already know.

Sebastian Moore, a teacher and theologian, tells about an experience of succumbing, discovering, and finally being

---

12. Mark Epstein, *Thoughts Without a Thinker* (New York: Basic Books, 1995).
13. Roberto Assagioli, *Psychosynthesis* (New York: Penquin Books, 1976).

freed from the tapes of the mind.[14] He was teaching a class that he thought was going very well. One day a fellow teacher told him that he had overheard some of Moore's students saying that they hadn't a clue about what was going on. This information flattened Moore. He went back to his room, "dead, destroyed, angry."

However, after a while, he began to ask what was going on here. Slowly he came to realize that it was not the information he had received that was causing him pain. It was the way he was processing the information. He was the victim of an euphoria tape in his mind. This tape programmed him to have "everything going splendidly or else I will resign." But this is not the way of actual life. The real situation is always that this student has understood and that one has not and that other one thinks she has but has understood something else. However, the mental tape will have none of this nuance, none of this actual way-of-things. The conditioning of his mind was blocking his entry into give-and-take of real life. Once he saw this, he refused to go along with the tape and returned to class energized.

This is the barest sketch of how some spiritual wisdom views the mind and its accumulation of knowledge. Perhaps one of the best statements of this overall approach comes from Rais El-Aflak.

Almost all the men who come to see me have strange imaginings about man. The strangest of these is the belief that

---

14. Sebastian More, *The Crucified Jesus Is No Stranger* (New York: Seabury Press, 1977).

they can progress only by improvement. Those who will understand me are those who realize that man is just as much in need of stripping off rigid accretions to reveal the knowing essence, as he is of adding anything.

Man thinks always in terms of inclusion into a plan of people, teachings, and ideas. Those who are really the Wise know that the Teaching may be carried out also by exclusion of those things which make man blind and deaf.[15]

This spirituality of mental alertness does not suggest adding anything. It encourages us to become aware of what is in the mind and to loosen our attachment to it. Often, it is our attachment to what we know that makes us "blind and deaf" to what we most deeply desire as it knocks upon our door.

Along every spiritual path, at one point or another, there is a need to set up a relationship with the mind. However, within health care settings a spirituality of knowledge seems particularly appropriate. A spirituality of knowledge would contribute significantly in three areas—issues of uncertainity and trust in doctor-patient relationships, dealing with organizational dialogue on key issues, and relating to the reality of deteriorating health in ourselves or our family or friends.

Daniel Sulmasy has noticed a strong intolerance of uncertainty in both patients and physicians.[16] They want precise knowledge in the present and sure fire prognosis for the future. Yet uncertainty is inherent in the process of diagnosis

---

15. Idries Shah, "Sufi Teaching Stories," in *A New Creation: America's Contemporary Spiritual Voices*, ed. Roger S. Gottlieb (New York: Crossroad, 1990), p. 109.

16. Daniel Sulmasy, *The Healer's Calling: A Spirituality for Physicians and Other Health Care Professionals* (New York: Paulist, 1997), pp. 23–36.

and treatment. He quotes Paul Ramsey, who wrote, "The function of medicine is not to relieve the human condition of the human condition." This failure to acknowledge uncertainty obscures the actual situation and undermines the trust that is central to the relationship between physician and patient. Sulmasy suggests a new toleration for uncertainty and with it a new configuration of the doctor-patient relationship.

Part of this new configuration would be that clinicians would begin to prioritize decision making over certitude and process over results. This new openness to not-knowing would naturally lead to a deeper trust, a trust in God, who also does not submit to the panicky human concern for certainty.

> God is the point of our hope, the context of our care, the source of our courage to reach out in uncertainity to love our patients—to care about them, to care for them, to think about them, to talk to them, to touch them, to heal them, to be with them through sickness and death and even, perhaps, beyond the horizon of the human into eternity. We can be certain of none of this. We can only have faith—faith enough to be healers for people broken in body and in spirit who entrust all their uncertainty to our care.[17]

This is an invitation to take seriously the not-knowing context of all our knowing.

If this new vision of medical care is appealing, how will it be accomplished? The drive for certainty in a fundamentally uncertain world is a tape of the mind, born of its fear and

---

17. Ibid., 36.

anxiety. Once we recognize this tape, we can resist its power to drag us along its unreal path. We can live in the real world, where knowledge is a powerful ally for better living and dying. But this knowledge is always limited and arises within an essential context of not-knowing. This realization keeps us from clinging to what we know and, paradoxically, stimulates our efforts to gain further knowledge. When we resist the tape of absolute certainity, we enter into a world of both knowledge and trust, the proper world for humans to inhabit.

The spirituality of knowledge can also contribute to organizational analysis and decision making. In his book on the learning organization, *The Fifth Discipline*, Peter Senge, following the thought of the physicist David Bohm, makes a distinction between discussion and dialogue.[18] In discussion, different views are presented and defended. The goal is to decide which view is the best and has the greatest chance of success. Most of the thinking is done before the meeting, and the success or failure of the meeting is determined by whether your plan won or lost. In dialogue, this is not the case. Views are presented in order to see something new. There is the expectation that the group may become open to "a flow of larger intelligence" (Bohm). The drive to decision making may have to wait upon a more complex and rich exploration of what is at hand. Senge believes both discussion and dialogue are needed in a learning organization.

However, discussion is "business as usual." This is the mode of communication that most organizations are familiar with and, in many cases, it is the only way people formally

---

18. Peter Senge, *The Fifth Discipline: The Art and Practice of the Learning Organization* (New York: Doubleday, 1990). pp. 238–239.

talk to one another. In the complex and ever-changing situation of health care, there may be an urgent need for dialogue. In dialogue, participants do not know the action-outcomes before the conversation. Actions are a by-product of dialogue. Therefore, there is a need to trust the process of talking. Indeed, there is a need to learn how to participate in a dialogue. For those skilled in debate and who always think in terms of winning, this is a new learning.

Bohm suggests that one of the skills associated with dialogue is the ability of participants to suspend their assumptions. People should be able to "hang their assumptions" in front of themselves and the group. It is here that the spirituality of knowledge enters. In order to do this, one has to both know the assumptive level of the mind and resist identification with any of its contents. Assumptions are not on the surface. In order to become aware of them, we have to engage in inner observation, an observation that is attentive and nonjudgmental. Once they are uncovered, we have to keep them "at arm's length" if we are going to suspend them. Any identification of ourselves with our assumptions results in defensiveness and antagonism. If these prerequisites for dialogue are crucial in a time when health care organizations either learn or disappear, then the spirituality of knowledge is a path for all, especially leadership.

The spirituality of knowledge is also important for how we relate to the health limits and losses we and our family and friends experience. Once I was walking into a hospital room to visit my friend, Frank. Another friend of Frank's was walking out. She grabbed my arm and led me away from the door. She whispered, "Wait till you see Frank. It's not him." When I went in and saw him, I knew what she meant. Frank was drained, in pain from the surgery, and had none of the spark I had always associated with him. But he was still Frank. He was just a Frank unlike the Frank I previously knew.

Part of the spirituality of knowledge is to learn to hold lightly the models we have of each other. The shock of seeing Frank in so un-Franklike a position was a testament to how the mind clings to past models. We cannot imagine a Frank other than the one we have in our minds. So we say, "It's not him." But, of course, it is him. It is the real Frank, not the Frank our mind is clinging to. This tendency of the mind to hold onto past models is also evident when we are the objects of our own observations. After some physical or mental setbacks, we bemoan, "I am not myself." Our minds are clinging to a past rendition of ourselves, and this clinging is keeping us from entering into the only self there is, the one living in this moment. One benefit of the spirituality of knowledge is that it offers a freedom to be in the present. When the mind resists being controlled by past and future tapes, it opens us to what is now.

Receptive meditation, selected memory, and cultivating not-knowing are practices that can keep us in this beneficial relationship to the mind and its knowledge. Receptive meditation is often called the Witness.[19] It means we pull consciousness inside and watch the flow of thoughts. We do not react to them but take up a nonjudgmental stance. This meditative practice reinforces our soul connection and slows the mind. It also gives us knowledge of the mind's content. If we persevere in this meditation, this inner spaciousness becomes part of our consciousness. We become facile at distinguishing who we are from what we are thinking, and we learn how to use our thinking to serve the deeper purposes of the self. Selective memory focuses on times when we have combined knowing and trusting, or experienced dialogue, or stayed present to a person even when our minds clung to an outmoded model of who they were. These spiritual experiences, like all experiences, had a beginning and an end. They happened and are now over. However, we can recall them and, when we are doing so, the inner space of those times returns to us. Then we know in the present what the proper relationship to knowledge "feels" like. With memory as a guide, we can reinhabit the inner space that proved so beneficial in the past. If we persevere in this process, the spiritual state of fleeting experiences can become a spiritual trait of everyday consciousness.

Not-knowing is a practice of entertaining the dark edges that surround all our luminous circles. It does not glory in what we know. It entertains all we do not know. Elizabeth Lesser tells the story about the North Indian classical singer Pandit Pranath, who would wander around the practice room saying, "Allah knows; I do not."[20] Cultivating not-knowing simultaneously renders what we do know more precious and relativizes it in relationship to what, at the moment, is still unknown. Not-knowing is a particularly helpful practice when dealing with the behaviors and motivations of people. It invites us to inquire rather than to judge. In many spiri-

---

19. Scholars often divide meditation into concentrative and receptive. See Michael Washburn, *The Ego & The Dynamic Ground* (Albany: State University of New York, 1988), pp. 141–43. For insights into the Witness, see Ken Wilber, *One Taste* (Boston: Shambhala, 1999), pp. 273–76.

20. Elizabeth Lesser, *The New American Spirituality: A Seeker's Guide* (New York: Random House, 1999), p. 34.

tual traditions, the wise are those who know that they know not.

A Spirituality of Compassion

We all have bodies; yet, at any given moment, some bodies are healthy and some are ill. We all have minds; yet some minds are first in the class and the corporation, and some minds are forever catching up or permanently left behind. We all have relationships and social position; yet some relationships are loving, and some are indifferent, and some social positions are important, and some are menial. We are all souls; yet some souls are conscious of their communion with the Divine Source and living in peaceful action, and other souls are unconscious of their connection to the Divine Source and struggling painfully with life. We are both separate and the same, isolated and connected to one another. Conventional perception stresses the separateness and isolation. Spiritual perception stresses the sameness and connection.

The realization of sameness and connection is the first step to cultivating compassion. When the Catholic Pope gets off an airplane in any country, he kisses the earth. He does this in every land for all the earth is sacred. There is a sameness to the different terrains of every country. Although many may think the earth of their country is sacred in a way the earth of other countries is not, this gesture tries to awaken another perception. When the Dalai Lama arrives in a country, he announces to all who are there, "Everyone wants happiness and doesn't want suffering."[21] This is true of all, so all are

---

21. Jeffrey Hopkins, "Equality: The First Step in Cultivating Compassion," *Tricycle* (Summer, 1999): 26–29.

bound together. Both the Pope's gesture and the Dalai Lama's sentence could be turned into profound spiritual practices. Although one may seem to be politically inspired and the other to be a throw-away line of a banal philosophy, they are both strenuous efforts to reverse separatist thinking. If you kiss with mindfulness the floor of every house you enter and say internally to every person you meet, "Everyone wants happiness and doesn't want suffering," you will be on a path of realizing your neighbor is yourself.

Some spiritualities see this perception of sameness and connection as a gradual deepening of consciousness. In the Middle Ages, Christians were encouraged to meditate on the mystical rose. The meditation began at the top of the rose where the tips of the petals do not touch. At this point they would realize the truth of separateness. Then their eyes would glide down the rose and rest on the overlapping sections of the petals. This sight would encourage consciousness to realize similarities and commonalities among what appeared as separate. When the eyes reached the base of the rose, all the petals came from the same stem. This was the deepest realization of the one source of all things and therefore a fundamental communion among all things.

Spiritual consciousness recognizes a fundamental communion within which separateness exists. When we are aware of this communion, it overflows into the experience of compassion. In the Christian gospels, compassion is the "engine" of three of Jesus' greatest stories. The prodigal father, seeing his son while still a long way off, is moved with compassion and runs to him (Lk. 15: 11–32). The Samaritan, seeing the robbed and beaten man in the ditch, is moved with compassion and goes down into the ditch to help him (Lk.10:25–37).

The master, hearing the plea of his servant, is moved with compassion and forgives him (Mt.18:21–35). Compassion is the inner energy of action—a welcoming action, a helping action, a forgiving action. In other words, in recognizing deeper communion, compassion overcomes separateness by embracing others in their needs.

Being in the presence of suffering is the classic experience that pushes perception along the continuum of sameness and difference, connection and separateness. To state the possibilities in terms of stark contrasts, the suffering will cause us to recoil or reach out, to become isolated or connected. In the presence of suffering—our own and that of others—we may become afraid, basically for our own life and well-being. Stephen Levine lays out the path of this fear: "When your fear touches someone's pain, it becomes pity." We pity ourselves and others. On the one hand, we wallow in "Why is this happening to me?" On the other hand, we shrink back and say with misplaced piety, "There but for the grace of God go I." Our suffering or the suffering of others does not bring us into the consciousness of connection and open the path of compassion. It pushes us into a heightened sense of separateness.

Although this may be the instinctive reaction to suffering, spiritual teachers point out that there is another invitation in the experience. The second half of Stephen Levine's observation is "When your love touches someone's pain, it becomes compassion."[22] In spiritual teaching, love is a meta-

---

22. Quoted in Sogyal Rinpoche, *The Tibetan Book of Living and Dying* (San Francisco: HarperSanFrancisco, 1994), p. 200.

physical condition before it is an act of the human will. When, through the experience of suffering and pain, we recognize the metaphysical conditions of our essential communion with one another, this realization moves us to compassion and we reach out. We find the love that is the grounding for compassion.

Sogyal Rinpoche has constructed a script out of many requests, a script we probably know only too well. "My friend's or my relative's suffering is disturbing me very much, and I really want to help. But I cannot feel enough love actually to be able to help. The compassion I want to show is blocked. What can I do?" Sogyal Rinpoche suggests a number of exercises to awaken love and compassion. All of them tap into, in one way or another, the connective flow of love that is the ultimate structure of reality.[23]

Recently, I was present at an event when suffering became the path to the realization of connection and compassion. I was working with elders on the possibility of late-life spiritual development. Every Tuesday for four weeks, eight people between the ages of eighty-two and ninety-two gathered around a table in the recreation room of a retirement living facility. The gender mix was seven women and one man. (Men are not long-distance runners in the game of life.)

The gathering was a sea of suffering. Walkers were parked next to a number of the chairs. The people began sentences with, "After my third operation . . . ." Strokes, heart attacks,

_____
23. Ibid., 193–208.

diabetes, arthritis, and various other maladies were part of the group.

These elderly folks came together at my invitation to explore the possibility of their spiritual development. They were interested, but occasionally I could catch a glint in their eyes or a shared look that made me suspect they were humoring me.

The background theory was that old age is a time of physical, psychological, and social losses. The body declines, aspects of the mind's functioning are not as sharp, and many relationships have been broken by sickness, death, and confinement. However, it may also be a time of spiritual growth. It may be possible to develop spiritually even while there is decline in other areas of life. So it says here.

I have always felt a major piece of spiritual development is wisdom. People realize certain spiritual truths. They see through the surfaces of life and into a deeper wisdom that frees them from various debilitating obsessions. Yet these spiritual realizations are fleeting. The point is to hold them in awareness long enough for healing to have a chance. I use stories from spiritual traditions to help this happen. The hope is that people will see and talk about their experience through the wisdom the story provides.

I tried a story from the Hindu tradition about the toughness of the human desire to heal suffering. It did not catalyze the group into conversation. I told a Christian story about God's presence in time of suffering. They smiled, but they did not talk.

The final story was a tale of a woman who lost her husband. She was inconsolable. The grief had lasted so long she felt she would never love and live again. Finally, she went to see a holy man. She entered his hut and told her tale. The holy man said he would like to help her but he is cold. Could she go around to the neighboring houses and gather some wood? They could make a fire and warm his old bones. Then they could address her grief. She agrees, but as she is leaving, he says to her, "Only take wood from a house that has lost no one."

Three women in the group said in unison. "She didn't get any wood."

I paused and finally said, "That's what the story says."

"But her grief lifted." This line, the actual last line of the story, came from a frail woman who earlier had asked us to pray for her husband. Recently, they had to be separated because his Alzheimer's had progressed to a point where he was uncontrollable.

Never at a loss for words, I said, "That's what the story says."

Then they talked. They all talked.

I sat back and listened.

I did not listen to one thing or for one thing. I listened to it as a whole. It had many notes, but a single piece of music was being played. It came to me slowly. When I saw it, it was obvious.

Suffering wasn't a problem for them. It was just what was. It was not an offense to be railed against, not was it an insult to who they were or something they feared and fought every waking minute. It was just what was there. And it opened them to one another in genuine compassion. Their common suffering made them one. And in a strange way, as in the story, they were healed. Their suffering did not go away, but their grief was lifted.

On the way home from this session I remembered a story Stephen Levine tells in *Healing into Life and Death*.[24] A woman by the name of Hazel was suffering with cancer and came into the hospital in "a very contracted state." She was angry and nasty with everyone. The nurses called her "a real bitch on wheels." Then one night when she was in fierce pain, she just let it all go. A series of profound realizations followed. She joined with what she later called "the ten thousand in pain." She joined with "a brown-skinned woman, breast slack from malnutrition, lying on her side, a starving child sucking at her empty breast . . . an Eskimo woman lying on her side dying during childbirth . . . the body of a woman dying by the side of the road after a car accident." Later she said she saw that her pain "wasn't just *my* pain. It was *the* pain." It is a terrible truth to tell—suffering often cracks our hardened heart and releases us into the world of suffering where all people at one time or another live.

This spiritual belief about a dimension of life where we are all in communion, and these stories that tell of times when people realize this truth need to be reinforced by practices. In general, practices should bring into consciousness the truth of our connection rather the surface condition of our separateness. I am always impressed by how spiritually developed people, who to outside eyes are holy and exceptional, always stress how they are just part of it all. For example, Bede Griffiths, a Benedictine monk who lived and worked in India for many years, always prayed the Jesus prayer, repeating at every chance, "Lord, Jesus Christ, Son of God, have

---

24. Stephen Levine, *Healing into Life and Death* (New York: Doubleday, 1987), pp. 11–13.

mercy on me, a sinner." He reveals his inner consciousness as he prays, "have mercy on me, a sinner."

> I unite myself with all human beings from the beginning of the world who have experienced separation from God, or from the eternal truth. I realize that, as human beings, we are all separated from God, from the source of our being. We are wandering in a world of shadows, mistaking the outward appearance of people and things for reality. But at all times something is pressing us to reach out beyond the shadows, to face the reality, the truth, the inner meaning of our lives, and so to find God, or whatever name we give to the mystery which enfolds us.[25]

His prayer reminds him, despite a lifetime of spiritual development, that he is one with everyone else, wandering in a world of shadows.

Another example of this sense of connection can be found in a remarkable reflection of Stephen Levine and others on their experience of working with a "cancer" patient named Katherine. She contacted their Dying Project and told them she had cancer. Over a period of time, she met with many of them and attended their retreats. Finally, people became suspicious, and it was discovered that she was "faking it." She was not ill. In fact, she had a history of faking sickness and abusing morphine. Eventually, she disappeared. Levine and his associates reflect:

---

25. Father Bede Griffiths, "Going Out of Oneself," *Parabola* (Summer 1999): 24–25.

Clearly, our work with Katherine as with all such beings is work on ourselves. Another teaching in helplessness, another opportunity to let go of ourselves, to be no one special, to gently watch the constant changes of the mind—going beyond hope and doubt until at last fear dissolves in the sense of endless being, in the connectedness that joins us all. Katherine's mind is no different from the minds of any of us. It was just that she held in fiery pain to her suffering. We can only wish mercy for such beings and for those parts of ourselves too that scream out for attention and in confusion rail against the way of things. Her suffering is as real as anyone's we have worked with. We wish her Godspeed.[26]

There are many profound observations in this reflection. But the recognition of sameness is one of the most startling. "Katherine's mind is no different from the minds of any of us. It was just that she held in fiery pain to her suffering. We can only wish mercy for such beings and for those parts of ourselves too that scream out for attention and in confusion rail against the way of things." It is this recognition of sameness that is the wellspring of their compassion. The title of the episode is "A Deeper Pain Than Dying."

How does the spirituality of compassion relate to health care?

From one point of view, human suffering is the center and foundation of the vast enterprise of health care. Every facet of medical knowledge and care is, in one way or another, geared to the fragility and vulnerability of our bodies and

---

26. Stephen Levine, *Meetings at the Edge* (New York: Doubleday, 1984), p. 189.

minds. Insurance coverage is built on a careful mapping of how we break down. Even the upper level organizational structures are concerned with patient satisfaction and so are continually reminded of the suffering at the center. Therefore, the whole health care enterprise lives and works in the presence of suffering.

This fact can be ignored by our fearful minds. But when it is faced, an invitation is issued. Either consciousness will harden into separateness or awaken into communion. If it awakens into communion, we will be moved by compassion.

And if compassion flows, all the issues and situations of health care—universal coverage, allocation of resources, truth telling in diagnosis and treatment, participation in clinical trials, compassion fatigue, unions, pain management, mergers, access to medicines, and more—will look different. How these situations will be specifically addressed in the future and how these issues will be concretely resolved cannot be foreseen. But the fundamental vision of connection and compassion is infinitely creative. It is infinitely creative because it is grounded in the infinite creativity of the Divine Source. Once we know we belong to one another in an essential way, we will not dismiss the challenge. We will find a way to walk each other home.

Conclusion

Although it is 6:00 a.m. and still dark, the parking lot of the hospital is already filling up. In an hour only the far lots will be available. People are filing from their cars and meeting up with others who are getting off buses. They are all moving toward the hospital, its many windows spilling light into the last darkness before the day.

Who are these people?

They are spiritual people who have come from spiritual communities with beliefs, stories, and practices that help them stay conscious of their spiritual depth and the spiritual depth of the situation. Although health care is a socially structured enterprise geared for the effective delivery of service, it welcomes the diverse spiritualities of people. It has many reasons for doing this, and the concrete procedures of spiritual hospitality are still being worked out. However, besides these background spiritualities, there are foreground spiritualities that connect to individual and organizational values and help implement them. They are beliefs, stories, and practices around the recurring health care experiences of self-remembering, knowledge, and compassion. These spiritualities are welcomed because they can increase the quality of human interactions. The hospital-medical center complex, spilling light through its windows, realizes the complementarity of the spiritual with the socially structured delivery of health care. It welcomes these people out of the darkness.

EIGHT INJUNCTIONS

□ □ □ ■

Injunctions have an honored place in spiritual teaching. We are told to do or not to do something. "Do not be afraid of that which can kill the body and do no more." "Do not identify with the fruits of your labor." "Know yourself." "Be silent and know that I am God." "Throw the bucket into the sea." "Honor your father and mother." "Love your neighbor as yourself."

Although there are many injunctions, there are not corresponding instructions. We are told what to do or not to do, but we are not told exactly how to do it or not to do it. For example, how does one go about not being afraid of the death of the body when the mind is filled with prerational tapes about how to protect our bodily identities at all costs? Or how does one go about disidentifying with the fruits of one's labor when wanting to be recognized for what we have done is one of our strongest driving forces? The spiritual texts are often silent about how to deal with these difficulties. This may be a regrettable lack of specificity on their part or it may be a deliberate ploy. Imperatives without instructions may combine to point spiritual seekers in a particular direction and yet allow them the surprise of discovering truth for themselves.

As we struggle to carry out the injunctions, we learn what we need to know. We encounter obstacles and allies both in ourselves and in our situations. We have to work with these blocks and openings, these resistances and desires. If we are patient and persevere, we will develop spiritually through this work. This means we will coincide with ourselves as spiritual people dynamically living in physical, psychological, and social reality. It also means our lives will become an invitation for others to undertake their spiritual adventure. All this can come about from following the injunctions. We come to see injunctions not as primarily goals to be accomplished but as paths to be walked.

In this spirit, I would like to suggest eight injunctions that flow from the exploration of health care and spirituality developed in the previous pages. These injunctions are scatter shot. Some apply more directly to organizational endeavors; others encourage individual efforts. Some might be attractive to patients, others to healthcare leaders, and still others to medical caregivers. As a whole, they are meant to initiate or continue the spiritual path of those who are interested and involved in the relationship between health care and spirituality.

1. Try to think and act in terms of the four dimensions—physical, psychological, social, and spiritual. These dimensions are both distinctive and mutually influential. The trick is knowing when to stress distinctiveness and when to stress mutuality. For example, the distinctiveness of each dimension means that activity and excellence in one dimension cannot substitute for lack of activity and mediocrity in another dimension. If there is high turnover on the nursing staff because of social-organizational changes, the response is not to initiate programs in nurse spirituality in the hope that it will offset the organizational crunches. Spiritual development does not make up for deficits in organizational design. On the other hand, the dimensions are mutually influential. For example, facial surgery is going to effect psychological self-image; mental peace is going to contribute to physical recovery; social reconciliation with a former enemy is going to open spiritual channels. Although the presenting difficulty may be in one dimension, it may be appropriate to work in the other dimensions with the hope of helping the whole person. Holistic care entails becoming familiar with the four dimensions and learning both how to pursue them independently of one another and how to integrate them into a holistic approach.

2. Connect grassroots spiritual advocacy with organizational initiatives. Often certain individuals within organizations see themselves as sensitive to the importance of the spiritual. Particular doctors, nurses, social workers, managers, or chaplains may have awakened to the spiritual as the permeating context of health care interactions. On their own they initiate efforts to recognize and respond more fully to the

presence of the spiritual. At the same time, the organization may be considering some sustained efforts to integrate spirituality into patient care or to provide opportunities for spiritual development to employees. The bottom-up efforts and the top-down directives should connect with one another. On the grassroots side, this means acknowledging the need for structure and working with people who are not fully sensitized to how essential the spiritual is. On the organizational side, this means both explicitly espousing values that legitimate the inclusion of the spiritual within the range of health care concerns and putting structures and policies in place that facilitate the spiritualities of people.

3. **Place spiritual needs within the larger context of spiritual development.** The conventional way of thinking is that people are spiritual beings and therefore have spiritual needs that should be met. Just as there are physical, psychological, and social needs, there are spiritual needs such as the need for worship, for forgiveness, for a sense of ultimate meaning. However, this approach may be too limiting. Spiritual needs arise in people at specific times and places and fit into the dynamics of their spiritual biography. The stories of people's spiritual journey are tales of advancement, stagnation, and regression. There are models of spiritual development that throw light on where people have come from, where they are at, and where it is possible to go. Every need arises out of a past history and opens into a future possibility. Once people are comfortable with including the spiritual in the range of health care concerns, the next step is understanding and discerning the unfolding of spiritual development.

4. **Create a climate that continually invites patients and employees to tell their spiritually significant experiences**

in story form. A spiritually significant experience is any happening that triggers spiritual awareness in a person. It is an event that opens one or both eyes of the soul, and, consequently, the person realizes the presence and activity of the spiritual dimension. The telling of the story is important because through the telling the experience establishes a place in memory. When memory hosts the fleeting experience, it holds it steady and moves it toward being a stable structure of perception. The spiritual experience contributes to spiritual growth. Also, one individual's storytelling invites other stories. In a round of storytelling, the reality of the spiritual is slowly acknowledged and accepted.

5. **Heed spiritual wisdom.** The religious traditions of the world, folk traditions, and certain movements in psychology articulate spiritual wisdom. They express in image, story, and discursive language what the spiritual is, how it influences all forms of life, how it is resisted, and how it is embraced. The more we nourish ourselves with this wisdom, the more we commune with the spiritual and appreciate its ways. If we are interested in the spiritual, it seems natural to explore the resources of the past and to listen to those presently among us who are more developed spiritually. Their wisdom cannot substitute for our own efforts at realizing spiritual truths, but they often illuminate brightly what we have only a glimmer of. They light the path we are walking along.

6. **Learn to appreciate the tension between organizational procedures and spiritual wisdom as the necessary forerunner of more integrated approaches.** Spiritual wisdom has a great deal to say about the same areas of life that organizational development deals with—competition, goal setting, creativity, perseverance, time management, motiva-

tion, roles, the use of authority, profits, and so forth. However, it is not immediately evident how the spiritual wisdom and the organizational wisdom mesh. For example, spiritual wisdom recommends silence as a way to deepen interpersonal communication and encourage creativity. Organizational culture often assumes silence is a weakness, a failure to see what to do, and, most importantly, a waste of time. Organizational procedures stress goal setting, time lines, and strategies to meet those goals. Spiritual wisdom is leery of too much emphasis being placed on the achievement of goals that have been previously set. In the pursuit of the goals, the emergent possibility of the moment might be overlooked. Organizational and spiritual wisdom are both needed. When both are worked with and held in tension, a new approach that integrates both wisdoms is possible.

7. **Try going within.** Most people recognize the importance of faith on their spiritual journeys. In fact, faith is often the permeating context of spiritual development. We begin a spiritual path because we put faith in a spiritual teacher or in a spiritual tradition. Faith sustains us in times of spiritual blindness. The ultimate mystery we enter into does not succumb to our clever efforts at control and so elicits from us faith in the form of trust. However, there is also the possibility of direct experience. We can become conscious of the spiritual dimension as the ultimate ground of our own personal reality and, consequently, as present in every situation. The path to this awareness is within. Every spiritual tradition encourages interiority. Through spiritual practices—such as meditation, prayer, silence, and retreats—we discover we are in communion with an infinite reality and with all things that are sustained by that infinite reality. As we cultivate this

inner awareness, we begin to balance faith with knowing. Now we live in the to-and-fro of knowing and not knowing, a to-and-fro that never ends. The personal experience of our inner grounding means we have experienced ourselves spiritually. It is no longer a matter of belief that can be eroded by argument, but a matter of knowing that deepens and is expressed in living.

8. **Try going without while remaining within.** When we go within, we connect or reconnect with the soul space. The soul space opens into Spirit, and it is the nature of Spirit to give itself. This self-giving of Spirit encourages a self-giving in us. Two traditional ways it does this is by illuminating the mind and inspiring the will. We understand the spiritual depth of situations, and we are impelled to act. The self-giving of Spirit does not replace our natural dynamics of knowing and doing. Rather it makes them more excellent, more complete, more attentive to all that is happening. Therefore, the task is to stay in touch with the self-giving Spirit as we give ourselves to the many tasks and duties of our lives. This process is aptly described as going without while remaining within. When we explore this human possibility, we begin to walk the path of incarnation, the struggle to make Spirit flesh.

C.P. Cavafy wrote a famous poem called "Ithaca," playing upon the classical reference of Ulysses' journey toward his home island. He suggests that the final arrival at Ithaca is not as important as the journey.

Ithaca gave you the marvelous journey.
Without her you would not have set out.

And if you find her poor, Ithaca won't have fooled you.
Wise as you will have become, so full of experience,
you will have understood by then what these Ithacas mean.[1]

In spiritual traditions, injunctions are something like Ithacas.
If you work faithfully with an integrated dimensional approach, if you attend to both grassroots and organizational currents of spiritual interest, if you steadfastly see spiritual need as a moment of spiritual development, if you listen to the stories of the experiences that have awakened people to the presence and the activity of the spiritual, if you search out spiritual wisdom wherever it may be found, if you welcome the mismatch of organizational and spiritual approaches as the tension of a new integration, if you practice going within to the soul room of your own house, and if you flow from that space without ever leaving it into the boardroom or the clinic or the work site or your sick friend's house or your own hurting body, then you will have become wise in the ways of health care and spirituality.

---

1. C.P. Covafy, *Collected Poems* (Princeton, New Jersey: Princeton University Press, 1992). p. 36.